GETTING REAL ABOUT SEX ADDICTION

GETTING REAL ABOUT SEX ADDICTION

A PSYCHODYNAMIC APPROACH TO TREATMENT

GRAEME DANIELS AND JOSEPH P. FARLEY

ROWMAN & LITTLEFIELD
Lanham • Boulder • New York • London

Published by Rowman & Littlefield
An imprint of The Rowman & Littlefield Publishing Group, Inc.
4501 Forbes Boulevard, Suite 200, Lanham, Maryland 20706
www.rowman.com

86-90 Paul Street, London EC2A 4NE

British Library Cataloguing in Publication Information Available

Library of Congress Cataloging-in-Publication Data
Names: Daniels, Graeme, 1968– author. | Farley, Joseph P., 1960– author.
Title: Getting real about sex addiction : a psychodynamic approach to treatment / Graeme Daniels and Joseph P. Farley.
Description: Lanham : Rowman & Littlefield, [2022] | Includes bibliographical references and index.
Identifiers: LCCN 2021042832 (print) | LCCN 2021042833 (ebook) | ISBN 9781538158043 (cloth) | ISBN 9781538158050 (paperback) | ISBN 9781538158067 (epub)
Subjects: LCSH: Sex addiction—Treatment. | Psychodynamic psychotherapy.
Classification: LCC RC560.S43 D36 2022 (print) | LCC RC560.S43 (ebook) | DDC 616.85/833—dc23/eng/20211103
LC record available at https://lccn.loc.gov/2021042832
LC ebook record available at https://lccn.loc.gov/2021042833

For Don, Michael, and Bill

Contents

Preface

When Graeme approached me about collaborating with him on a book project, I became excited. After all, our friendship goes back nearly 20 years, and I know him to be a thoughtful, very smart, and generally fun guy to hang out with. As he's already written several books, I felt honored that he was seeking my input. We have had some great discussions, so I thought the cross-fertilization of ideas would be stimulating. We met at a local diner to discuss the project over breakfast. When he told me he wanted the book to focus on the psychodynamic treatment of sex addiction, I got a bit nervous but didn't share my apprehension until the first draft was nearly complete.

My anxiety about participating in writing a book on sex addiction increased over time and I hadn't told anyone but immediate family about it. It finally came up in a discussion with a friend who was visiting from out of town. When she casually asked me what I had been doing lately, I spilled it and noticed my anxiety as I monitored her facial expression. I felt like the 13-year-old hiding a pornographic magazine under my mattress, except it was a book. I had several reasons for concern. First, I didn't consider myself an expert in the field of sex addiction treatment, but perhaps I should. Gladwell (2008) says doing something for 10,000 hours makes you an expert at it, and I have conducted approximately 10,500 sessions with sex addicts throughout my 35-year career. I have a general private practice in Northern California, which is my primary source of income. Each week I see 30 to 35 patients and supervise students. About 20 percent of my patients suffer from what I would call sexual addiction, for lack of a better term. About 50 percent of my patients suffer from disorders of the self, commonly referred to as personality disorders. The rest are what you might call neurotics; many suffer from anxiety or depression, and some are adjusting to a recent, very difficult life-changing event like the death of a family member or the loss of a job. About 30 percent have experienced severe trauma and are suffering related effects. You may have noticed that these percentages don't add up to 100. That's because someone can have a personality disorder and severe trauma. This is often the case.

Second, I was afraid of being known to the community as a sex addiction therapist, of becoming a "therapist of perverts." I worried that coming to my office might become like entering an adult bookstore, where you look around twice before you get out of your car to make sure no one sees you before you enter the building. I didn't want every patient I saw to suddenly become guilty by association. Imagine the man who comes to me for treatment because he's been feeling depressed. He's working hard in therapy, but some days he can barely get out of bed and make it to his appointment. One day his wife, bored and curious, searches my name online and finds a book about sex addiction. Making an a priori assumption that her husband has been living a secret life all these years, she starts calling divorce attorneys. (You can see my vivid imagination at work.) Now, my patient is not only coping with his depression but has to cope with his wife's anger, suspicion, and unrelenting questions as well. In my worst fantasies (yes, I do that), the private practice I have built over 30 years evaporates, because no one wants to see the guy who treats sex addicts. I become a divorced (oh, yes, my wife leaves me too because she thinks I must be a sex addict), homeless therapist with a scarlet letter. My colleagues avoid me like the plague, so I add loneliness to my list of afflictions. (Some of you are laughing, but those of you who work in the field of sex addiction can probably relate.)

A colleague of mine, Don Mathews, founded the Impulse Treatment Center (ITC), a clinic focusing on the treatment of sex addicts and their partners. It is the largest outpatient clinic of its type in North America. At any one time, it is not unusual for Don to facilitate 15 groups of six to eight men simultaneously, all of whom are seeking treatment for problematic sexual behavior. In addition, he usually runs about four groups for their spouses. Many of these men come to treatment because their partners discovered that they were acting out sexually. I wonder if many of them looked over their shoulders when they entered the front door of the ITC for the first time.

Unlike ITC patients, most of mine come to treatment without that scarlet letter. Some of the partners of my patients are aware of their problematic sexual behaviors, but the majority of the men I treat for compulsive sexual behavior are living with their addiction in the shadows. Many come to treatment for another reason, like depression or problems at work, and not until later does it become apparent that they are engaged in compulsive sexual behavior. This is a secret that is not given up easily. It may take years to build enough trust in the therapeutic relationship to support the telling of this secret.

I hope that helping to write this book does not create undue stress for my patients, those with sex addiction and those without. It may not be considered professional in our field to talk about this, but I am quite fond of many of my patients, both male and female. I really like them. Sometimes, I even love them. Early in my career, I wouldn't say that. I was so concerned about doing my job right that I didn't allow myself to really hear my patients, much less form an attachment to them. I didn't have enough life experiences to appreciate what they were going through. As I've gotten older, I find myself appreciating my patients more and more.

The Personal Psychotherapy of the Therapist

Several years ago, I was going through an especially self-critical moment in my own therapy, when I was feeling like the worst person on earth. (I have sat with many of my patients going through similar moments.) It was toward the end of my treatment, and we were discussing termination; I made a comment something like, "I'm sure you will be relieved not to deal with me anymore." Part of me believed it, but I protected myself by saying it jokingly. She saw right through me instantly. (We therapists can be some of the most difficult patients, and I'm sure that I put my therapist through the wringer a time or two.)

She looked at me with the kindest, most compassionate look on her face and said, "Don't you know that I adore you?" I was floored. I didn't know how to respond. It took my breath away. On the drive back to my office, I remember thinking for the first time that she didn't have very good boundaries and wondering if she was having erotic countertransference to me. I was starting to question my relationship with my therapist, for whom I had developed a great deal of affection and respect. Later that day, I looked up the word *adore*, and discovered that it means "to love and respect." As you can imagine, the focus of our next session was that simple sentence, which affected me so profoundly. As I write about it, it still affects me. It affects not only the way I see myself but also the way I see my patients. It is as fresh to me today as it was at that moment.

I remember looking at my schedule of patients for the following week. How many of them did I adore? How many of them did I love and respect? I have not yet dared to say to any of my patients what she said to me that day, but maybe someday the moment will call for it and I will respond in the only honest way that I can. I certainly do adore many of the patients I see every week.

This book shares with you some of the research about the lasting impact of psychodynamic psychotherapy, one of its distinct advantages over psychotherapy based strictly on cognitive behavior (Shedler, 2010). I have internalized the relationship I developed with that therapist and feel that its impact on my life continues to grow even though I no longer see her. In reading psychotherapeutic literature, what I find most useful are easily comprehensible descriptions of theory accompanied by illustrative clinical vignettes. Good authors do this well, and this is what we are striving for.

We also appreciate a sense of humor, and nothing can be more humorous than taking a step back from a ridiculous situation and appreciating the complexity of the human condition. The antidote to bottomless despair about a predicament is to appreciate the hilarity of it. Yes, it's a means of self-defense. Because we're rather cowardly, we don't share examples of the many ways in which we can make fools of ourselves, which we do regularly. Sharing foibles with close friends allows us to laugh together, but the idea of readers laughing at us doesn't seem like much fun. In fact, it seems horrifying.

Our solution to this dilemma is a cowardly one. We tell you about the human condition through the experiences of our patients. Isn't that convenient? Isn't that what we do when we write a clinical book? We describe someone else's experiences to save ourselves a great deal of shame and embarrassment. According to Bering (2013), each person has their own deviant sexual quirk, which would be sure to turn their face red if exposed. We certainly don't want this for ourselves or for our clients, so we have tried to be respectful of our clients and the predicaments they struggle with. We make every effort to change identifying information and details so that if our patients were to read this account they wouldn't recognize themselves. That's always our goal when sharing vignettes, either in writing or in person. Without confidentiality, therapy is ineffective.

In addition to finding humor in the human condition, I find a great deal of inspiration in it as well. The courage of my patients is often bewildering, and I find myself inspired daily by their struggles and perseverance in situations where I would have folded. I feel deeply honored to be able to support myself in a profession in which people let me into their lives at their worst possible moments. I get to see and understand things that are much more amazing and inspirational than any work of fiction. In the book, *Working*, by Studs Terkel (1974), the author recounts opportunities to speak to people who do jobs I could never imagine. One worker, a stonemason, described in detail the care and artistry with which he chooses the right stone for the right place. I get to do a version of what Terkel did. Along with the dreadful situations that bring each of them into therapy, I get to hear about my patient's lives and details of their vocations, and I get to share all of that with you. I have worked with (mostly not sex addicts) surgeons, emergency room doctors, dentists, researchers, appliance repairmen, attorneys, politicians, professional athletes, contractors, software engineers, civil engineers, mathematicians, police officers, accountants, insurance agents, hospital administrators, filmmakers, realtors, psychiatrists, nurses, oral surgeons, city administrators, owners of manufacturing businesses, electrical engineers, property investors, loan officers, social workers, psychologists, marriage and family therapists, high school and elementary school teachers, firefighters, paramedics, graduate students, and high school students. It's an inspiring list. And those are just my patients from the particular week I wrote this paragraph. If I were to list all the professions represented in 35 years of work, the list would be long, but nowhere near exhaustive. I've never worked with a herpetologist, but there is still time. It's on my bucket list.

The engineer describes the anxieties that keep him up at night after a structure collapses in Kansas City and lives are lost. The young software engineer working on artificial intelligence in the medical field describes his passion for the work and what he hopes to accomplish in the years ahead. The plumber, who commonly drives 150 miles a day in some of the worst traffic in the United States and is the one the other technicians call for advice, juggles his schedule to make his appointment in between five customer visits scattered over the Bay Area. These are my heroes. We often comment on how enviable a position that we occupy is. We get to listen to our patients tell their stories of love and work. In what other profession would we be granted this privilege? This book is an expression of gratitude for what we do and who we serve. May we always live up to the trust that has been granted to us.

Acknowledgments

From Joe Farley

To my father, John, who taught me how to be a man. To my mother, Mary; wife, Susan; and daughters, Kaitlin and Emily, who taught me how to relate to and respect women. To Jerry Schwartz, my dear friend who taught me how to be more human. To my friend and colleague Don Matthews, who taught me most of what I know about the field of sex addiction treatment. To James Masterson, who taught me how to be a good therapist and who encouraged me to show up with my real self. To my elementary school friends who strangely still enjoy my company and whose names I have appropriated and assigned to the clients I have written about in this book. To my friend and colleague Graeme Daniels, who extended the generous invitation to cowrite this book with him. To my Friday morning men's group, John, Jon, Graeme, Ben, Don, and Bob. You are the elders who have taught me about life and brotherhood. You have taught me not to be afraid of other men.

From Graeme Daniels

I'd like to thank my coauthor Joe Farley for his good humor and patience, plus the curiosity that inspired the idea for this book. I'd further like to thank the following teachers, mentors, and colleagues for their influence and support, recent or over years, and for thinking with me: Caroline Andrew, John Kravitz, Brian Needleman, Dave Borof, Joan Gold, Paul Kramer, Ben Jones, Jon Colladay, Shelly Nagel, Kathryn Furst, Joanne Shurter, Jonathan Keeley, Maureen Katz, Georgine Marrott, Ken Seider, Lara Weyland, Pedro Job, Samuel Chase, Mitch Wilson, and Don Mathews. Thanks also to the many clients of ITC and to my patients in private practice.

Thanks as ever to my parents and to my wife, Maria.

Introduction

What Are We Wearing?

By now it's a tired joke to ask whether sex addiction is real. For the quick benefit of analytic readers, this use of the word "real" is not Lacanian (signifying the ineffable), but it is expressive of something plainly truthful. Real or not, the condition known as sex addiction (or the related terms sexual compulsivity, hypersexual disorder or hypersexuality, "out of control" sexual behaviors, or the not-quite-synonymous "problem sexual behaviors") is treated alongside more widely recognized conditions, like anxiety and depression disorders and chemical dependency. Sex addiction is treated in hospital settings, in specialized group homes, and in the formats of individual, couples, and group therapy in private practice offices. It is often aimed at the wealthier members of society who, like others, continue to ask, "Is this really a thing?"

Still, addiction is a serious matter, and treatment of it became an institutionalized mandate with passage of the Affordable Care Act, which required all insurers and state Medicaid programs to pay for alcohol and substance abuse treatment and extended coverage to an estimated 32 million Americans. But insurers will not pay for treatment of conditions unrecognized by the medical establishment. Since sex addiction is measurable but is not a diagnosis in the United States, sex addiction treatment remains a boutique service or is treated under the guise of another diagnosis. Having produced numerous books on the subject, sex addiction advocates promulgate a few standards to practitioners and consumers for the treatment of sex addicts and those impacted by their behaviors: specialist credentials; wide use of assessment tools; and protocols of intervention across elastic stages of a developing disorder.

This book is not so much an instruction as an inquiry, and maybe an idea as to how to talk, write, and think about psychotherapy. Our purpose is not to promote sex addiction as a concept, much less to extol its leading models of care. Our perspective is peripheral to the supposed front lines of sex addiction treatment, the high-profile residential facilities that we won't name specifically. Are such programs analogous to needle-exchange clinics or detox centers? Not really. Meanwhile, private practice psychotherapy is where disclosures of sexual misconduct are often first heard, yielding referrals to intensive short-term programs that may include medical components. Or private offices may be where sex addicts land after those intensive interventions are over.

Our vantage point is that of most psychotherapists. We observe the ubiquity of sex and addiction in our culture; the increased accessibility to porn and prostitution; and the intersecting issues of sex, gender, trauma, and violence. Of course, increased accessibility has enabled appetites that previously might have been contained. But how were such habitual sexual behaviors described or categorized before the term addiction became so saturated with meanings? Repetitive sexual acts may have been called womanizing or nymphomania. And what about the repetitive use of pornography or sex offending behavior? The terms perversity or libertinism were once invoked to represent predigital–era porn use, pedophilia, or paraphilia, to indicate behaviors that were nongenital, harmful to children, or unconventional. Terms like pedophile, satyriasis, Don Juanism, and nymphomaniac recall epithets like dipsomaniac, which was used before alcoholism was identified as a progressive and fatal disease.

We dodge expert-like assertions about terminology, choosing instead to review literature and offer illustrative vignettes, plus a touch of mischief. Since the naming of the issue is a matter of opinion, we generally choose the term sex addiction, though more often refer to "acting out" to indicate behaviors (not necessarily sexual) that unconsciously replace words, memory, thought, and feeling to give the concept a psychoanalytic meaning. Our stance is intended to steer away from preconception yet maintain that sex addiction is real insofar as it exists in psychic reality, as a defense against affect. In other words, the concept represents not just behaviors, but wishes—conscious or unconscious conflicts that are real to the afflicted patient and which merit analysis. If that doesn't seem like a simple or straight answer, know that we won't give many straight answers. We're here to provoke thought, not impose it, and to examine the thoughts of others, especially as revealed in terminology. Terms like addiction, trauma, acting out, betrayed partner, or perpetrator are used to frame a therapeutic episode. Prefixes like poly, di, and bi are used to exhibit fresh thinking. In contrast, the prefix mono betrays rigid positions, flat-earth ideation. Regardless, most terms are presented to consumers in a biased fashion, steering thought with words just as we intend with ours.

In this text we use terms like consumer to indicate distance between an idea and its adherents, and concepts like circularity to indicate redundancies or unfalsifiable or preconceived logic. In addition, we alternate references to patients and clients (using the latter more typically in a couples or group format); therapist and clinician (and sometimes analyst); and to the pronouns *he* and *she* (though *he* is more often represented). We refer to object relations (OR) theory or psychoanalytic theory when conceptualizing but use the umbrella term psychodynamic to indicate method. Also, though we are trained practitioners of the disorder of self model devised by James Masterson and will give a sampling of his method, no singular model or theory is being manualized or promoted here.

Our intent is not to confuse you, but to make a point: Those who present for treatment are subjected to (and sometimes absorb) the jargon and other linguistic norms of professionals, but their experience may have little to do with intellectual content. Some patients are quite sensitive to language. Understandably, many who seek help do not like being subject to terms like addiction, and they like it even less when the label is attached to the topic of sex, regardless of whether appropriate assessment tools are used. Others seem hungrier for diagnosis and assessment and appear to thrive in a treatment atmosphere with a tight intellectual structure and a directive air. In keeping with a spirit of caution, we also make use of deliberately equivocal terms like "would-be sex addict" or "self-identified" sex addict. These terms mirror the position we ordinarily take when people present for treatment. We take seriously the nature of problems, but we do not assume a defined condition. So sex addiction, as both a concept and an assessment designation, is treated here as an open question.

Amid questions of diagnosis and assessment arise matters of metapsychology; moral inquiry; notions of religious, Aristotelian, or Kantian virtue; and the psychoanalytic concepts of transference and countertransference. Therapists like to view themselves as nonjudgmental, nurturing of the shame-faced and the traumatized.

Our offices are refuges, places to be honest in an atmosphere of emotional safety. Truthfully, however, we observe that the field of sex addiction is laden with value judgments and recommendations with uber-ethical underpinnings, even though their sources and targets are often disguised. Though biases may vary regionally or subculturally, we think the overall voice of sex addiction treatment is not dominantly religious or conservative or antisexual, but rather progressive and tolerant of sexual diversity. Contrary to what may be popular opinion, professional objections are aimed at deceit, not promiscuity or unconventional sexual practices. The near-categorical imperative of therapy is truthfulness—speaking truth despite fear, shame, or guilt. Objections are reserved for the exploitative and the entitled, not necessarily the unfaithful or spiritually disobedient. Criticism of religion as an enabler of sexual neurosis may speak to the upbringings of many self-identified sex addicts. However, it also colludes with a latter-day subterfuge: while organized religion gets tagged as a source of moral judgment by both professional and lay observers, we think that social justice is the reigning moral lens of sex addiction treatment.

This contrarian observation alludes to our book's title, which reflects loaded marketing in the field of sex addiction treatment: virtue signaling with promises of redemption for the wayward, justice for victims, or veiled hate for religion and the man. We virtue signal with our titular claim of honesty: a warm regard for the men and women we treat juxtaposed against a pitiless scrutiny of ideas. Truly, if this book is a critique of treatment models, it's not because we think sex addiction doesn't exist or that many standard intervention strategies aren't worthwhile. However, we think that social and consumer-driven assumptions skew treatment approaches.

About our information-gathering: we have read and we have listened. For years, we have read books on sex addiction, and while our text is not quite an exegesis of this thinly studied field, we offer a range of opinions about its flagship literature. In addition to scholarly articles (the must-reads of psychoanalytic or attachment theory), we have read popular works, including blogs and articles published in commercial magazines. Why? Because, like it or not, sex addiction is now embedded in the public imagination. We have also consulted—and sometimes argued—with colleagues about these subjects at workshops, networking events, and conferences such as those presented by the Society for the Advancement of Sexual Health (SASH). Further, we've spoken to and listened to many patients, men and women beset with a spectrum of sexual problems. The result of all that talking, reading, and listening is poured into this text, yielding accounts of what happens in our offices, and what we think is happening in the offices of other therapists.

Full disclosure: as coauthors, we have not only shared our thoughts as colleagues, but as friends and members of an ongoing men's support group. Our shared experience in an emotional risk-taking circle of men was one of the primary reasons for writing this book together. We owe a debt of gratitude to this group, and in particular to ITC founder Don Mathews, a man impressed with ideas and persons but not institutions, who has provided a cat's eye view of sex addiction treatment over the last twenty years.

Over a parallel stretch of time, we have come to know each other's thoughts. Knowing each other's defenses and tender spots, we understand how and when to confront issues and when to tread carefully. We talk seriously about sex and addiction, and about crossover topics like trauma, gender, and personality, and sometimes we stop talking seriously and have some fun instead, like anti-homophobic teasing. In the process of writing this book, we call each other and ask, "What are you wearing?" before posing some thought-provoking topic.

Beyond our conversations, we think that men and women struggle to speak of these matters with one another. Therefore, we often suggest that they split into separate sessions or groups, similar to our men's group. We advocate for group therapy, specifically group therapy in which men and women meet in separate quarters, because in many cases it seems better for a group of men or a group of women to figure stuff out among themselves than strain to explain themselves to members of the opposite sex.

The following pages illustrate episodes of individual, couples, and group therapy. The latter is a common format in the treatment of addictions, reflecting what Sigmund Freud (1921) once wrote about group psychology: that identification facilitates emotional ties within a group, reflecting herd instinct, suggestibility, and the avoidance of difference. The theoretical lens of this book is psychodynamic, which is hardly the norm in the field of sex addiction treatment. However, our vernacular and insights shouldn't be obscure. While the label of sex addiction continues to strain for medical legitimacy, many will think that nothing is more addictive than sex, and that a diagnostic category pertaining to it is long overdue. In psychoanalytic theory, Freud presented a foundational idea over a century ago: the mind apparatus lives with the tension between two principles, pleasure and reality. Pleasure in the id leads to displeasure in the ego. In a repressed yet organized mind, instincts toward sex and aggression are meant to be contained by a strong ego, girded by a third structure, the superego. Hence civilization and common discontent. Later, Arlow (1987) may have linked addiction with trauma when he opined, "Play is used to master traumatic experiences. When play takes on a compelling, obsessive quality, it is no longer play" (p. 33). Dissociation, a state of discontinuity often brought on by trauma, seems to sever links between mental structures. Feelings like guilt and shame are split-off and rendered unconscious; contrary to social expectation, they are not integrated, but experienced separately. Those not prone to addictions often do not understand this phenomenon of the addictive mind, and self-identified addicts tend to think they never will.

Explanations of psychoanalytic theories pervade this text alongside illustrations of psychodynamic theory and Mastersonian method. What you might glean from the case illustrations is our attention to unconscious process and relational knowing: an attempt to stir thought about self and other. Although it might not seem controversial, the approach isn't necessarily popular. Indeed, when we have presented portions of text to early readers, we have received critical feedback. Sex addiction represents behavioral problems calling for a directive approach featuring behavior contracts, accountability systems, collaborations with collateral contacts, and social support. Some argue that the deepening, esoteric thoughts of analytically oriented method are contraindicated.

We contest several assumptions that such arguments contain. The first one is that psychodynamic approaches ignore the need to confront acting out behaviors. The second is that deepening approaches proscribe concurrent use of auxiliary support systems like group therapy or 12-step program involvement. For example, the psychoanalytic model of Masterson outlines an approach that addresses behavioral acting out (a "testing" phase) before proceeding to a "working through" phase, which may include support systems throughout treatment.

In some respects, we conform to sex addiction treatment norms with our own reified approach, and with the relative absence of at least one psychoanalytic pastime: attention to dreams. That said, this business does often feel like a dream in which the opposite of what is happening is said to be happening. On the whole, critics of analytic approaches seem to think that sharp demarcations exist between phases of stability and instability, and beyond that, between points wherein feelings can be explored versus times when they can't. They regard treatment as a linear, stage-oriented process, not an intersubjective or dialectic happening.

Additionally, we offer that assumptions about class, religion, and (especially) gender contaminate treatment strategies, and while we generally refer to men and women in a heteronormative context (because that's the dominant context in our practices), we do so with modest apologies. But the larger issue here is the ironic "post-truth" concept of narrative that strains data, espousing facts that are then spun into dubious conclusions. As clinicians, we are inclined to think about—but not know—the cultural influences on interpersonal and intrapsychic function. Knowing (versus knowledge) is elusive. Though abstractly agreeable, a stridently politicized faction in and outside psychoanalysis asserts that psychotherapy has existed over time within a sclerotic patriarchal and capitalist culture, and that observations of individuals should be filtered through that piece of knowledge and altered by reactions to it. Because dominant factions of society aren't known for lamenting hate or disadvantage that is directed at the other, this sound-biting counterculture explains the following phenomenon: Ask "what is misogyny?" and the average man or woman will know the word's meaning and have something to say. Ask instead "what is misandry?" and at least 8 out of 10 will likely guess that it's an online video game or a character in a Netflix sci-fi series.

The filmmaker and philosopher Susan Sontag (1973) wrote that our economic system requires nonstop entertainment, especially the mass consumption of images, to anesthetize injuries of class, racism, and sexism. According to this view, the exponential growth of pornography is just one example of overabundance masquerading as freedom. Meanwhile, images depict masculine vigor and hoary notions of feminine reserve, while others represent female sexual empowerment. The latter may counter-objectify men but otherwise simply vacate male sexuality, creating space for feminine display rather than sexual interaction. Trending discourse sells revolution and subsumes individuals under protean identity norms. Such discourse intersects with matters of sex and addiction, yielding broad, proprietorial commentary. You can almost hear the diatribes across office walls, even in private practice settings where collegial water cooler conversations are fewer. These colleagues of ours, who like to pretend that they're still outnumbered, toiling in the margins, are saying something like the following: We're here in numbers, recruiting more as time passes, and our conscience is the new superego.

This conscience inclines sex addiction advocates toward humanistic or systems theory, which serve as pretexts for social commentary, as well as more concrete interventions typically directed at sex addicts. We depart from these approaches, thinking them reductionist and (as manifested in the demographics of sex addiction treatment) obsessed with a critique of masculine ego. This "sex addict" is subliminally hateful, but also hated, and is right to be wary of caustic voices. Sex addiction specialists who say they "work within a system" usually mean interviewing other family members and including them in sessions, thinking the addict is a straw man for whom reality-testing, limit-setting, and overall progress rely on the input of reliable witnesses. The moral imperative behind this approach is the adverse impact of addiction on significant others.

However, what is ethical about a treatment that isn't truly the patient's idea? The systemic approach justifies heavy-handed tactics like the insistent use of polygraphs, or overcommunication between professionals to reconcile accounts, because treatment in this context is a bit like an investigation. We think this does not protect confidentiality and therefore does not generate fuller disclosures, much less a deeper, longer-lasting understanding of underlying problems. For all parties, the dialectical tension is between needs must and hypothesized capacities for changed behavior and consciousness. The process is one of perpetual duress, tethered to an external mandate and utilitarian aims. Or, it breaks away, carving an uncertain space for the mind of the one.

The cognoscenti in the sex addiction field also think of sex addicts as narcissists who may want help but find it difficult to ask for help. They also want approval, and the secret behind the "not asking for help" cliché is that approval is even harder to ask for.

Women are tagged less often as narcissists, and in general, female sex or love addicts are treated differently, less numerously, or with less dogged pursuit. While some fumble with sociological theory to explain this phenomenon, we offer the following: as providers, we play by different rules when we work with women. Our examples include reports from other providers, featuring snatches of interventions about which they seem proud, including confrontations of "live" objectifying behavior and the "calling out" of sexual innuendo and other provocative gestures by men that raise their ugly heads in treatment. That is not the problem. However, in the current professional climate, which has been dominant for some time, if we were to sit in a group of six to eight women (or one-on-one with a self-identified female sex addict) and "call out" provocative dress or flirtatious or seductive and therefore treatment-resistant actions, we'd be accused of misogyny or of "traumatizing" a vulnerable patient and might soon be defending ourselves in court or before a licensing board. In contrast, although a female therapist may not care to rebuke the provocative, sometimes even masturbatory behaviors of male subjects, she can do so with relative impunity.

While we operate from the sideline of private practice, we are not impervious to the influence of culture or hegemonic systems. During the COVID-19 crisis, the needs of systems and individuals seem more symbiotic than ever. This has compelled psychotherapists to adapt frameworks—such as telehealth, with all its distancing and privacy-reducing flaws—to new norms. While the lasting influence of the COVID-19 phenomenon is unknown, we begin our text with a more historically prevalent pattern—an impacted-partner driven therapy—that precipitates many sex addiction treatment episodes. Such episodes are shaped by observations of trauma. This is not because rates of posttraumatic stress disorder (PTSD) diagnoses are highly comorbid with assessments of sex addiction or impacted-partner experiences. Actually, we barely allude to data on such phenomena, because trauma is not just a feature of psychiatric diagnosis. It now denotes a metapsychological standard across professional or algorithmic messaging: An inextricable link between trauma and psychopathology, which at times can render the concept of trauma diffuse, or even banal.

We further notice pushback against so-called co-dependency models of treatment to explain and treat impacted partner responses. Whether this theoretical shift is ethical or merely trending, it emphasizes the premium placed on patient accountability. The discovery of addiction dislodges the theorized symmetry of fault between members of a warring couple. The addict is responsible for his problem behaviors—no arguments there. The arguments lie at the intersection of addiction and relationship problems. In the context of addiction, what responsibility do impacted partners have for relational conflict?

Besides such questions, we also look beyond the office walls, with opinions about sex (activity, not biological type), gender, ideology, mythology, poetry, art, and even the lesser art of pornography. Fair warning: this book contains passages that conjure explicit porn and violence, followed by analysis of their themes. Why? We tire of reading opinions that pontificate about porn by authors who pretend they never look at it. Beyond that controversial subject, the elephants in our subtext are the loose indices of gender equality (such as sexual freedom and wage equity), and those phenomena of inequality that remain largely syntonic with the collective ego: the asymmetrical role of women in the physical care of children and the expectation that men perform society's more physically rigorous or dangerous jobs but exercise physical restraint when in conflict with women. Thus, our discussion is a minor subset of a broader conversation that seems perennial and never-ending, yet somehow barely begun.

In this barely conversant, sexually, and otherwise dystopic mood of 2020–2021, we talk about justice, and about not-so-common discontent. We wait for a vaccine, fight wildfires, invest in technology (something called 5G), or—more regressively—plywood, and hope that all the smoke, storms, riots, and lies soon abate. People talk. But they don't really listen. Against this backdrop, the identified (typically male) sex addict is an unlikely pariah in some respects. He is sometimes a top dog, or a runt running from hate while a not-as-but-still guilty pack scrambles for privacy. He is an unreliable witness, a reporter of suffering, who speaks of sex as a need and its absence a privation. But his onlookers aren't necessarily better witnesses. If this view renders our approach ambiguous, a reactionary agitation that will marginalize already marginal authors, then so be it.

We're here in lesser numbers, pirates on an open sea, violating cultural gag orders currently aimed at our demographic, and we think that this book will tease out readers' biases because in any model of treatment for people who have a problem relating to sex, you must ask yourself, who is the treatment for? Who or what is it meant to serve? An individual? A system? A community? Also, if this is not a zero-sum game (as some put it), or a war on those who declare war (who in turn insist that their rivals declared war first), then where are the circles in our minds taking us?

CHAPTER 1

Trends and Norms in Sex Addiction Treatment

> Ah jeez, not this thing again. Why? What did I do? Name me one thing that I've done?
>
> —The character Fuchs, from the HBO series, *Barry*

Over 100 years ago, Sigmund Freud wrote that his patients' neuroses derived from their sexuality. He fashioned a model of mental health care in which patients were encouraged to speak their thoughts and feelings in an atmosphere of sexual and relational abstinence. That abstinence pertained to sexual behavior, not thinking about sex. The thinking was encouraged.

The term sex addiction was coined over 30 years ago as some observed a cultural obsession with sex that was both conscious and not. Regardless, it was damaging lives. This spawned a niche field within mental health that included doctors, therapists, and moralists with different views, all saying something at once new and old about sex.

Meanwhile, we don't talk that much about sex. Hypothesizing a change, Fonagy (2008) used computer-assisted word frequency analysis to study the number of terms about sexual body parts, sexual orientation, or sexual behaviors that appear in psychoanalytic literature. He found that interest in psychosexuality has declined over the last few generations.

CASE ILLUSTRATION: RICK AND ANNE

Shrugging seems like an innocuous gesture, a meaningless roll of some muscle north of a shoulder socket that is not connected to thought or procedural memory—just habit. In our work, we're generally more interested in interior lives than physicality, but we've noticed many such expressive flinches, these ridding actions of the body-psyche. A person's words fill time and therapeutic space, but they don't inform or provide insight, nor are they moving, for the words aren't really theirs. We think this true of men like Rick.

> The motivation for care isn't *his*. Because his words aren't moving him it seems like an act, like he's keeping the couch warm for someone else. These things that Rick's been asked to do—to speak words that explain past actions and then choose the right behaviors in the present and future—are not happening. His father, and his father before him, always said that actions speak louder than words, even important phrases like "I do." Rick considers actions, which he substitutes for words, to be more important, more reliable. Yet words have become important, especially now that his actions have let him down, disgracing him like they disgraced his father. Negative patterns repeat and keep repeating.

We are therapists. Specifically, we practice psychoanalytic psychotherapy, sometimes called psychodynamic therapy, a field distinguishable from classical psychoanalysis, though related. We do something. Or rather, we say something after a spell of listening, which does something that isn't easy to measure. Actually, our thinking about what we hear and see is more important than the words we say or the actions we prescribe.

As therapists, our thoughts aim at things like Rick's shoulder movement and convey our fascination with the unconscious: that reservoir of forgotten or hidden thought that creeps around body and mind, carrying the weight of many things, not just sex. The mind holds aggression, gentleness, envy, generosity, shame, creativity, guilt, gratitude, and love.

> Rick looks up quizzically, wondering what his latest therapist will provide. Leaving his thoughts, he questions where this therapist's thoughts are. What will therapy achieve? What problem will it solve? And how will it help him navigate the

> difficult evening that lies ahead of him? Will he manifest the progress of this therapeutic action by hearing his wife, Anne, like he hasn't done before? "Validate" her feelings like he has never done before? His therapy is meant to serve her needs as well as his own, but it would be easier if this were a report, like a spreadsheet of figures he could send to a bottom-line-craving boss. If he could just present data showing Anne what happens in these sessions, he might relieve some of the pressure he's feeling (and not feeling). If he could just assure her that everything's fine and that there's nothing more to worry about, then maybe she'd be happy. Then he'd be happy. She's not happy and hasn't been so for years. She has been especially unhappy in recent months, after discovery of a certain problem, first discovered on the household laptop and soon after on his smartphone. It turned out that this problem had been going on for years.

Discovery is a conceptual term in the field of sex addiction. It refers to the point when sex addiction becomes a known problem. That isn't really when sex addiction becomes a problem—it just seems that way because discovery confers reality upon previously disputed events. That thing: it exists. It happened. Infidelities and other sexually acting out behaviors may have been happening for years, but only emerge "in reality" after such discoveries, say, during couples therapy. After her discovery, Anne used Rick's laptop for a "healthier" purpose: to research treatment options relating to addictive behaviors, sometimes referred to as problem behaviors, out-of-control behaviors, or compulsive behaviors.

> The websites that gave Anne hope described worthy principles: accountability, boundary-setting, and relief from shame. The hard sell was in the stock footage on the site headers: the sorrowful look of a handsome man with his head in his hands, appearing bereft and regretful; an "after" picture of a couple frozen in fully clothed frolic, poised to resume love and intimacy now that a dark chapter of their lives is behind them. The latter image sold Rick on the idea, giving him some hope, although he kept that—like most of his thoughts—to himself. Without stating it explicitly, the images and rhetoric of this treatment program suggested that freedom from compulsion, shame, guilt, and whatever else was just weeks or even days away. It just took a phone call, plus a credit card.

At the end of his treatment program, Rick was told that he had a brain disease. Recommendations included polygraph exams to support his accountability and an aftercare plan comprised of individual therapy, possibly couples therapy, and 12-step meeting participation, all coordinated by professionals. After "not clicking" with two of the follow-up therapists, he began psychodynamic therapy. With me.

Rick comes home after appointments shrugging his shoulders in response to Anne's questions, saying he doesn't quite know how to explain what's happening, only that whatever is happening won't happen overnight. He's correct. I had mentioned that complex resistances interwoven with treatment would take time to unravel. Anne replies to Rick that this is not good enough, that it isn't serving her needs, and that he has not changed. She says that it's like traffic school: Rick has attended class but he keeps speeding, and then, when he's pulled over, he simply says he's going to traffic school as if that should suffice to absolve him.

Anne remembers talking to me during a phone consultation a week or so before their first couple's session (now a distant, fuzzy memory) and two weeks before transition to Rick's individual treatment, "as he is the one with the problem, after all." She'd done the reconnaissance work: made all the original calls; sounded out the approach, style, and philosophy of treatment; discussed the niggly issues of fees; and asked whether there was any chance that insurance might cover sessions if the issue was represented with discretionary euphemisms (sex addiction doesn't exist as far as insurance is concerned). Diagnoses such as anxiety or depression might be good enough for reimbursement but aren't nearly good enough for Anne. To her, concepts like anxiety, depression, and addiction are excuses for the trauma and betrayal that she has experienced.

During that phone consultation, she asked after the treatment approach. How long would the program take? Were there homework assignments to be completed by her husband between sessions and then returned for inspection and feedback? According to the program they had attended (for a month) and the books she'd been reading, these were standard recovery tools. I deflected the first question, indicating that my "program" was ongoing, as in not time-limited, and

> that it wasn't a program but therapy. I then asked whether she had ever been in therapy. She replied that she'd been one time. What did that mean? A single session? When pressed, Anne admitted that the episode had been brief. It became clear that intimations of a lengthy process were not satisfying, and so she found me evasive, equivocal, and unsupportive. "What are you, my nutritionist?!" she exclaimed. "It's like I'm having a heart attack and you're telling me to eat more apples and jog every day." She continued: "I've been through hell and back on this already. I need to hear something that will work soon, not a year, two, or like fifty from now!"

There is an insidious premium placed on words like soon or *now*. The latter is complicit in addictions, has assumed an immovable position at the center of consumerist society. It exists, rather ironically, in our latter-day systems of health care, including systems of mental health.

> I replied, unequivocally, that Anne might want something that will still work in two years, or even fifty. My conviction stilled Anne's complaints, leading her to listen more and remonstrate less. A plan was outlined: continued use of a support system—like a 12-step group—and meetings twice per week for a minimum of 90 days. Rick's behavior would be monitored insofar as I would remark if he wasn't disclosing. Honesty would be encouraged as he processed thoughts that had likely become separate from his emotional core, which is what happens when a person develops an addictive habit.
>
> I added that I don't give advice, because when people are told what to do they may comply or rebel, but all too often they stop thinking. Eventually, Anne seemed to understand that treatment wouldn't be like dog obedience school; her husband's failure to sit on command wouldn't constitute generalized failure. He might stall or at least diminish the acting out behaviors (actually, this happens often in early treatment, so some interventions are like placebos). He might establish a baseline of honesty with her about past transgressions; an agreement about what might be shared between them as they move forward. She might think of this as "setting the bone" before deepening the process, employing an awkward, dog-like metaphor that other professionals have used. (The mind is nothing like a bone, I think.)

In taking calls like the one from Anne, it's easy to get pulled into the pain of a betrayed partner and make promises hastily. Those involved can either be slow to respond, or too quick to placate the angriest or most desperate party, usually the person who has only recently discovered the problem or was previously in denial. However, note that when the offenses are personal—when they pertain to sex—denial is not a palatable vocabulary. It implies that a person exhibiting this defense is doing something wrong, or that they are inattentive, neglectful, or possibly stupid. Instead, the word trauma, taken from a Greek word meaning "wound, is often assigned to the developmental histories[1] of both acting out and nonacting out partners, and connotes victimization or survival rather than wrongdoing. Instead of being pathological in a shame-inducing sense, trauma is blame-reducing, implying something that needs be endured, like a disease. As a survivor of another's irresponsible behavior, the partner of an identified sex addict is afforded a little moral indignation, allowed a well-spring of anger, and assumes the right to direct efforts to rectify deeply rooted problems like addiction.

So, what is addiction, anyway? It's an open question, really, and across societal strata it seems we can't quite decide whether the term is derogatory or sympathetic. There are plenty of definitions out there, with diffuse meanings linking addiction and sexual disorders, and others involving compromised psychiatric language. One category within the American Psychiatric Association's *Diagnostic Standards Manual*, 5th edition (DSM-5), "Sexual Disorder Not Otherwise Specified," likely wouldn't cut it with consumers. Seriously, imagine being told that you have a "Not Otherwise Specified" mental health condition. Regardless, after 90 days or so it's not uncommon for an angry spouse of a husband, cast as philandering or else porn-obsessed, to demand more than a semantic understanding of conditions, specified or not.

Like many impacted partners, Anne wants observable changes, such as a melting of the defenses that are blocking

---

1. Building on Freud's (1905) postulate that the latency period (ages 6–12) involves unparalleled repression of sexual desires, Hunt and Kraus (2009) collected research indicating that child sexual abuse, which includes having a child witness a sexual act, leads exposed children, especially males, to adopt sexually inappropriate behavior, resulting in sexual dysfunctions (lack of sexual arousal, erectile and orgasm disorders) in adulthood.

> Rick's contrition. She's not satisfied with his wooden efforts to understand the feelings of a formerly trusting wife. Eager for truth and offended that Rick's newfound openness has yielded little more than calls for a renewed sex life ("I'm telling you how I feel, like you asked"), Anne threatens to pull Rick from what she perceives as an ineffective therapy and install him in another structured program that will do what his original program recommended: give decisive instruction and accountability via repeat polygraph exams, then offer penetrative therapy to elicit honesty, self-reflection, and appropriate guilt.

Intensive treatment educates participants about the impact of addiction. For a betrayed or impacted partner, it also facilitates a genuine, thorough taste of perpetrator empathy through something called a full disclosure exercise. In truth, this exercise will answer only some of her questions. Best of all in Anne's view, with each party's permission, an intensive treatment program will enforce honesty agreements authorizing the provider to inform nonacting out partners and collateral providers if and when the would-be addict slips in his behavior, or "acts out."[2] Rick's previous program applied this kind of agreement, for about a month. Why only a month? Because that's about as long as most such programs last.

> "I can't do it anymore," Rick said during one session. At this point he'd been in therapy for about two months, first in the intensive program and then over the last few weeks with his latest therapist: me. It wasn't clear what "it" was, much less that he'd actually been doing "it" for months. It was clear that "it" pertained to the relationship that existed before and since the discovery of his acting out pattern. Rick didn't think of himself as an addict, just a guy who made mistakes. He

2. As variations of the term "act out" appear throughout this text, its pedigree bears explanation. Freud (1914b) explained that the patient remembers nothing, but expresses himself through action, and repeats it through transference. Building on this idea, and observing that patients do not experience a whole-object transference at the outset of treatment, Masterson (1981) used the term "Transference Acting Out" (roughly synonymous with "acting in") to denote a range of behaviors that replace words and memory, and that manifest in treatment in defensive interactions, or what Jacobs (1986) termed reenactment.

insisted that he no longer made those mistakes. "The empathy. I could do it at first because I did fuck up. I fucked up a lot. But she doesn't recognize her part. She never has." Rick continued, indicating that he couldn't really empathize with someone whose thinking is flawed, whose feelings are grounded in distortions, and some of whose complaints aren't valid. I challenged his overwrought assumptions about the victim role, which he seemed to consider interchangeable with the role of perpetrator, by asking him some pointed questions. "Were the accusations directed at him untrue? Was the ongoing suspicion and distrust unwarranted?" "No," Rick conceded gingerly. "But what is the point of behaving (abstaining?) now and into the future if I get no credit for improvement, no real forgiveness?" In other words, what is the point of changing if his reputation remains frozen in infamy? Rick wanted his apologies and promises to end all discussion, believing that action, like thinking, terminates feeling. Rick's dilemma at once blocked mourning of what he'd lost and consigned that mourning to an abyss. I suggested that the decision to terminate thinking and feeling was his "part."

The background in such cases is often littered with childhood exposure to sexually explicit behavior (live or via media), and episodes of exploitative or secretive sex, covered up by a strategy of obfuscations, lies, or postponable truths that become as habitual as the sex acts themselves. Discovery of this pattern marks a turning point. The onus of proof shifts from accuser to accused, and from that day forward, the presumption of continued guilt lies squarely at the feet of the acting out person. The nonacting out partner has had her world turned upside down; she has suffered anxiety and humiliation that had previously been dismissed. Now that the problem of sexual behaviors and gaslighting[3] have been

---

3. *Gaslight* is a 1938 play and later a film about a man who torments his wife by lying about his behavior and disappearances as he searches for jewels to steal from her attic. (The lights in the attic dim the lights elsewhere in the house—hence the title.) The term has come to mean someone who deliberately seeks to induce anxiety, even psychosis, in another through deception. Interestingly, the play recalls Sandor Ferenczi's (1933) famous concepts of "identification with the aggressor" and "confusion of tongues": a sign of trauma is the subject's identification with and induction into patriarchy—an internalization of its demands—exploiting a child's dependence and need for love.

exposed, she assumes the moral high ground and the right to assess all efforts at repair.

Couples therapy in this context is not so much couples therapy as individual therapy plus consultation with a disgruntled spouse or partner. Patronized or matronized like an expert witness, the partner's pronouncements carry psychic equivalence, in which feelings equal facts. To reject or even equivocate over her accusations is unempathetic, and heaven forbid that redemption-seeking perpetrators (or therapists) would ever lack empathy.

> Rick complained that his wife kept moving the goalposts of reconciliation. "And she can't even see the goalposts," he added sourly. Addressing an earlier question, he insisted that he was able to self-motivate and had been this way all his life. He explained the sequence of expectations thrust at him. First, he was to cease sexual acting out behaviors, and then he was to commit to therapy. This seemed reasonable, so Rick complied with treatment for a while, at the same time mentioning that he thought his wife also needed help for a chronic, unidentified mental health condition. During his few sessions, he expressed guilt for pursuing an affair, shame for visiting prostitutes regularly, and even more guilt and shame for binging on porn because he associated that habit with losers. He expressed additional guilt for failing to keep all of this secret. At this point Rick reiterated this contrary point, recalling the regret he'd expressed about secrecy when he and his wife first met in my office together: "I never wanted to hurt her." He reviewed the evidence of his actions, plus the failure of his secrecy. His pattern begged a question, the sine qua non of addiction, according to many: *Am I in control?* "I can't win," he concluded morosely, not quite answering. Rick's use of a popular sports/competition metaphor stirred my associations: the peculiarly American emphasis on winning and losing outcomes. Some sports tolerate the implicit justice of endings without conquest.

Therapist: What about a tie?
Rick: What do you mean?
Therapist: You make it sound like you have to *win* something. Words like surrender and phrases like "keeping the peace" came to mind. This is your marriage. Ties, or a tie, is about coming together. Does anyone win, as you put it?

Compartmentalization, keeping separate what is considered good and bad, has a pedigree in psychoanalytic theory. Think splitting. Of course, this habit is not exclusive to so-called addicts. People organize and manage their feelings as a matter of normalcy. Addicts seem adept at this at first, and then not so much. As their problems progress, the compartments collapse or leak, and then all the secrets spill out, exposing the feelings of the troubled individual that were there all along, only buried. Then another problem begins: cleaning up the mess, gathering up the soiled underwear; riding the luck of near misses (discoveries) like Indiana Jones dodging that giant boulder. The idea is for unacceptable aspects of the self to be kept hidden so that a false self is protected while a whole self remains undiscovered. A secondary purpose is to protect others from what will prospectively hurt *them*. This consequence is often cited as the primary disaster when discovery inevitably occurs. According to Riviere (1936), the "seek a cure for others" position staves off unconscious guilt (Freud, 1923), yielding negative therapeutic reaction, which thwarts receiving real help for the self but enables superficial cooperation in treatment and a seeking of punishment for contradictory acts of egotism. Linked to the problem of hurting others (and the fear of being hurt), guilt is redeemable via conventional gestures—including apologies and forgiveness—which seem represented across cultures and transform guilt into remorse. Shame seems more deeply embedded and therefore blocks the relatively advanced state of guilt. Bly (1990) wrote of shame: "the sense that you are an utterly inadequate person on this planet, and probably nothing can be done about it" (p. 189). As a result, shame is hidden and can seem inaccessible. It silences the tongue, blocks efforts at repair from all sides, and can even make thought itself disappear.

Anne was devastated by the discovery of Rick's acting out history. In her scrambling to restore order she has manifested what some consider a version of PTSD. In psychiatric terms, PTSD features alternating states of hyperarousal and dissociation, accompanied by overreactions and under-reactions, which serve as regular, unpleasant reminders of a problem and of a former lack of awareness. The latter has left Anne feeling foolish for not knowing about the problem earlier. Rick seemed mostly aware of her first reaction (hyperarousal), especially as he faced daily interrogations about everything from his cell phone and credit card records, to the reasons for slow or nonresponses to texts, to a late homecoming after what he'd insist was simply a long and involved workday. Losing patience, thinly aware of his needs, he complained that he was tired and stressed and yearned for a loving, understanding wife, not an inquisitor.

Rick's tendency toward compartmentalization, intertwined with his sexual acting out, reflected a habit of split-off (denied, or "not me") feeling. "I'm doing well, managing to take my mind off things (stressors)," he said during one session. He imagined himself following accepted social prescriptions, sometimes echoed by professionals: Take your mind off your problems; don't overthink. He didn't understand the psychoanalytic task before him: to put his mind *on* things (reflect on them more, not less), and then to feel something based on that thought. Rick needed to think but not indulge and learn to tolerate the feelings that emerge. Unfortunately, his attention to his inner life was as barren as his empathy for Anne and others.

Where Sex Addiction Fits in the Mental Health Industry

You may wonder if sex addiction treatment is really like this, or if it's like this very often. Well, it's hard to say how much the previous presentation represents those seeking treatment for the loosely defined conditions addressed in this text. Sex addiction, or sexual compulsivity, is defined by Kalichman and Rompa (1995) as an "insistent, repetitive, unwanted urge to perform specific acts often in ritualized or routinized fashions." Twenty years ago, well-publicized academic literature suggested that between 17 and 37 million people were sexually addicted (Carnes, 2001; Cooper et al., 2000; Wolf, 2000). More recently, Woehler et al. (2018) estimated that sex addiction affects up to 6% of the adult population.

On the one hand, the conceptualization of sex addiction has seemed predestined; the only surprise is its relatively late arrival in the modern psychology lexicon. Freud regarded addiction as a displacement of masturbation, one habit substituting for the other (Gay, 1988). However, Freud might have thought the term sex addiction redundant, or a shorthand, indicating habitual failures to postpone pleasure, followed by self-reproaches. He would have described aberrant behaviors like voyeurism as perversions and would have described those somatically afflicted by sexual disturbances as hysteric, suffering from conversion disorder.[4] Later, the concept of repression will have covered everyone else for whom sex ever lurks in the unconscious. Unlike the common neurotic, the addict does not postpone pleasure to safeguard or even enhance its later experience. He or she seems unwilling to delay gratification, or else believes that it is not commonly available.

Although 12-step programs relating to sex or love addiction have existed since the 1970s, sex addiction–specific models of treatment have been around for roughly 30 years. The most widely known model is that of Dr. Patrick Carnes. According to his model, a sex addict uses sex as a mood-altering experience, suffers from a brain disease plus an intimacy disorder borne of a traumatized history, and is saddled by core self-beliefs that isolate individuals who privilege sex as their most important need. Carnes (1989, 1991) further suggested that recovery from sex and love addiction would require 5 to 8 years of treatment, suggesting a long-term treatment approach.

At a glance, Carnes' model would seem to fit Rick's need, save for the long-term prescription. Rick seemed disinclined to spend anything close to five to eight years looking seriously at himself, much less pursuing a recovery program intently for that period. To be fair, few if any of the programs Rick and Anne had researched on the internet suggested a commitment to long-term treatment—at least, not one that was structured, directive, and professionally led. From our perspective, the treatment approaches commonly advertised on websites seem reductionist. They serve as directive, promissory responses to anxious consumers, like the man who has been caught with his pants down doing that which he won't—or can't—stop doing, or the woman caught unawares by discovery of said behavior who scrambles for awareness, chomping at the bit for quick understandings and measurable change. "Do something about him!" He might make quick pronouncements and promises while he bites his nails, knowing that some part of him doesn't care

4. A term that is less prevalent in contemporary psychiatry, conversion refers primarily to neurological symptoms that don't have any anatomical explanation. Examples include seizures, numbness, and paralysis such as that of Anna O., a famous pseudonym for a patient of Joseph Breuer. Conversion is distinguishable from psychosomatic illness, in which symptoms like ulcers result from recognized anxiety.

about the treatment but rather wants more, and not just more sex but . . . more *what?* Still, wanting to restore peace he will submit to assessments and expert recommendations in early intervention. She wants answers, some weaning of his glandular excitements, and an antidote to his generally wayward mind.

Everything seems clear at the outset of a program: the bad behavior must go, and a clean slate made. The proposed action is twofold: (1) cease or diminish the negative behaviors that are causing harm, and (2) move on with an honest understanding of the past and present. Sex addiction problems don't typically emerge the way that substance abuse or gambling problems do. However, the criteria for sex addiction as promulgated by the Carnes model are similar to the criteria for dependency outlined in the DSM-5:

- Repeated failure to resist sexual urges or behaviors
- Engaging in sexual behaviors for longer periods than intended
- Excessive time spent engaging in sexual behaviors
- Excessive time spent preparing for sexual behaviors
- Engaging in sexual behaviors instead of occupation or social obligations
- Increasing frequency or intensity of sexual behavior to achieve a desired effect (i.e., tolerance)

With substance abuse problems involving dependency, a series of events leads to treatment, and a culminating medical or legal crisis (such as an arrest for a DUI) commonly leverages a help-seeking motivation. Physiology, including tolerance phenomena and withdrawal syndromes, is assessed when an afflicted individual presents for care, and potential medical problems are outlined and managed. Legal consequences may have already occurred but may worsen if the person seeking help doesn't take the proposed intervention seriously. Beyond detoxification, a person may be prescribed medication to stave off drug cravings, like Naltrexone in the case of alcohol, or Suboxone to ameliorate withdrawal symptoms of opioid dependence. Twelve-step group participation is generally recommended because of its abstinence-based focus and emphasis on fellowship with others who are similarly struggling. According to 12-step philosophy, aside from physical or legal problems, emotional and spiritual isolation are the long-term consequences of a progressive disease.

Addiction is a cultural construct, so its meaning is less codified. The profile of a would-be sex addict might seem to mimic some dependency patterns, but it seems to involve even more isolation. Also, the onset of a crisis is less dependent on a legal or medical event. Some clinicians and consumers rely on a medical lens to determine whether a habit merits treatment. However, the significance of a medical diagnosis may be more important financially than clinically. Inclusion of an assessment label within the DSM-5 or pronouncement of a disorder by the World Health Organization (WHO) has currency with insurance companies and other funding sources, allowing treatment to be subsidized by third parties. But this will support sex addiction treatment only if sex addiction achieves medical legitimacy.

In the meantime, would-be sex addicts often get in trouble with the law, and some even progress to the socially undesirable category of sex offender. Also, while sex addicts may suffer medical consequences, such as contracting sexually transmitted diseases, the biological argument for sex addiction is not based on the medical consequences of risky sex per se, but rather on an observation that addictive agents like sex operate under the control of areas of the brain in which pleasure-seeking and pain avoidance are activated. The neurons of the nucleus accumbens, amygdala, and hippocampus of the midbrain affect emotional regulation and memory. When released by midbrain neurons, the neurotransmitter dopamine produces feelings of pleasure, even euphoria. In addition, through functional MRI technology, Voon et al. (2014) have shown that the amygdala, anterior cingulate, and ventral striatum are more active in the brains of the sexually compulsive than in those of control groups. This mirrors findings relating to substance use disorders, suggesting that drugs like Naltrexone might be effective in reducing compulsive sexual urges. Lastly, orgasm produces dopamine surges much like those produced by cocaine and heroin. If repetitive, dopamine activation can modify the structure of brain circuitry, leading to adapted responses such as the development of tolerance and cravings (Carnes, 1991; Ikemata & Panksepp, 1999; Linden, 2011; Weiss, 2013).

Hypersexual disorder, a term proposed to the American Psychiatric Association for inclusion within its latest *Diagnostic Standards Manual* (DSM-5, 2013), consists of numerous criteria, all featuring the words "excessive" or "repetitive" (Reid et al., 2013):

- Excessive urges, fantasies, or behaviors that interfere with non-sexual goals
- Repetitive urges, fantasies, or behaviors in response to stressful life events or dysphoric mood states
- Repetitive engagement in the same habits despite the risk of physical or emotional harm for at least six months

There you have it: a condition that resembles the profile so often described, formally proposed for inclusion in DSM-5, but ultimately rejected. Note that researchers draw a link between a pattern of behavior and an afflicted person's emotional life (specifically, negative mood states including anxiety, that a person may evacuate or anesthetize through repetitive pattern behavior), and further, that this finding has been supported by other researchers (Bancroft et al., 2003). The factor of excess was originally identified by the WHO. That body's international classification of diseases (ICD) once included a diagnosis of Excessive Sexual Drive. The ICD-11 includes a health problem designated as Compulsive Sexual Behavior Disorder (CSBD), and characterizes the problem as "persistent pattern of failure to control intense, repetitive, sexual impulses or urges leading to repetitive sexual behaviors" (WHO, 2019), which sounds similar to the Kalichman and Rompa (1995) definition. So, research affirms that sexual arousal activates the limbic system and provides physiological and psychological rewards, but whether excessive arousal indicates addiction is ambiguous. The point of equivocation in our field is that many things are rewarding but not necessarily addictive. The insistence that "rewarding" and "addictive" are synonyms risks diluting the meaning of addiction. It focuses excessively on the agents of affliction (like sex or drugs) rather than a marked alteration within the mind. So, as far as medicine is concerned, the question of whether sex addiction exists remains open. This has research implications because, if our field doesn't standardize the condition, then it can't properly gather subjects to study, which means we can't credibly form conclusions and insist that our treatment methods are effective, much less anything like a gold standard. This leaves sex addiction experts in an awkward though not unique position, claiming to use evidence-based models of care while still proselytizing the condition's existence.

Because sexual activity is essentially healthy behavior, some psychotherapists and doctors argue that it shouldn't be thought of in terms of either dependence or addiction at all. Blevins (2016) assembled considerable research linking sexual behavior to positive outcomes, contesting what he thinks sex addiction specialists assert: that too much sex or too much of the wrong kind of sex is unhealthy or implicitly immoral. To contest the first point, he offered an exhaustive list of studies showing that enjoyment of sex is linked to greater life longevity and reduced instances of coronary disease, type 2 diabetes, endocrine diseases, and breast and prostate cancer. Furthermore, he cited studies indicating that an active sex life improves sleep and pain management (including migraines, menstrual cramps, and chronic pain).

In his book, *The Myth of Sex Addiction*, Ley (2012) went a few steps further. First, he contested the assumption that pornography is degenerating society by pointing out that sexual violence is half (statistically) of what it was in the early 1990s, and that teen sexual activity has dropped by 7%, while the use of condoms has increased by 16%. Ley disputed the rationale for hypersexual disorders, observing that they emerge from consumer and provider demand instead of research and that vague and subjective criteria is applied, echoing a critique by the British Psychological Society that the DSM-5 pathologizes normal behaviors, ignoring their social and relational contexts. Ley (2012) further argues that language is important. He points out that words like "moron" and "imbecile" were once clinical terms, with objective meanings that were subsequently lost due to popular usage. So, we should be careful with the word addiction, not merely trade on it or frame a treatment episode based on a popular point of reference.

To us, the complaints of skeptics like Blevins and Ley seem fair, if still presumptive. For example, the agents that elicit habit-forming behaviors may not necessarily be toxic in an intrinsic, medical sense. Addictive is not necessarily synonymous with destructive. Such criteria are subjective. That said, would it console a betrayed partner to know that a significant other's repeated cheating might help deter prostate cancer? Does the self-identified porn addict who stays up all night watching one clip after another, compromising his academic or occupational life during the day, take comfort in thinking that his overall sleeping habits have been improved by his obsession? Using the criteria of those looking to protect the image of the agent, food addiction would not exist because food is a necessary substance. But what about food that lacks nutritive value, such as processed foods, which spike insulin levels? Outside the medical realm, workaholism wouldn't exist if work were only deemed virtuous and useful. The cautionary chestnut, *too much of a good thing*, would have no meaning. In short, addictions would only matter if they were medically dangerous or morally suspect.

Sometimes ignored in the principled "sex positive" argument, or among other sex addiction skeptics, is the presentation of pleasure-seeking behaviors that continue despite negative consequences that are meaningful to those engaging in the behaviors. Zitzman and Butler (2009) offer the following counter-critique: "Resistance to using the term addiction is perhaps more a reflection of cultural sexual liberality and permissiveness than any lack of symptomatic and diagnostic correspondence with other forms of addiction" (p. 212).

It seems to us that insufficient weight is given to novelty-seeking or sexual boredom as factors in an acting out pattern. It's not so much that acting out to kill boredom is itself unhealthy. It's that acting out habitually—subconsciously, repetitively, without awareness of its secondary purpose, or against one's conscious wishes—is problematic. Although standardized thresholds of addiction are difficult to establish due to moral relativism or selectively applied ethics, the determination of addiction ultimately seems personal. Why? Well, one reason is that assessment of mental health problems needn't always be standardized. That's what's unique about the paradigm of psychotherapy. It makes the dissembling and problem-solving cycles of a supposedly addictive pattern complex. It calls for flexibility, patience, and the willingness to forego a rush to judgment, be it positive or negative. Psychotherapy represents the consideration of intertwining factors that are biological, religious, social, personal, interpersonal, and even ideological in nature.

The watershed event that precipitates a call for professional help may be inconsequential in medical or legal terms. It will likely not meet the criteria of an accepted diagnostic category, but the discovery by an impacted spouse or partner often marks the divide between a pattern behavior that is problematic but under control, and a problem behavior requiring professional intervention. This view echoes an observation by Corley and Schneider (2002, p. 43), but we would highlight the contrast between the treatment-catalyzing events of sex addiction and those of chemical dependency even more. An alcoholic or a drug abuser might enter a program because his or her spouse discovers a stash of contraband, but this is less typically a decisive event in problem assessment. By the time a drug abuser is ready for treatment or at least compliant with a treatment mandate, the fact of their drug use has generally been known by others for some time. In that context, the progression of frequency, related symptoms, or negative consequences (legal, medical, monetary, or academic) are the focus of concern. When a would-be sex addict enters treatment, it is often because the discovery of the behavior, whether or not it has been perennial or compulsive, is brand new. The secret of a sexually acting out pattern tends to be guarded more assiduously by the acting out person. Even presumably nonjudgmental peers don't hear about sexually addictive behaviors nearly as much as they do about substance use or substance abuse. Therefore, its seemingly careless revelation tends to be more indicative of lost control by the afflicted individual and is more of a shock to that person's partner.

Because sex is so much more personal than drug use—seeming to evoke more shame and guilt than perhaps any other aspect of human life—sexual acting out tends to evoke stronger feelings of betrayal or inadequacy in nonacting out partners, not to mention moral disgust. Clinicians who work with families affected by substance abuse or dependence often observe a sense of frustration, weariness, and incomprehension. Parents of adolescents may experience feelings of inadequacy, thinking that the child's disorder is an indictment of poor parenting. This can also be true of partners of an alcoholic or drug addict. They, too, may present for treatment feeling exhausted by efforts to help their loved ones.

However, the reactions of parents, partners, and spouses of alcoholics don't rival the ferocity of betrayal, shock, and humiliation often presented by a partner of a purported sex addict. In the aftermath of discovery, there is little room for negotiation with partners as to controlled use, or anything like harm reduction, with respect to sexually acting out behaviors, whether it be porn use, online or live affairs, or the use of professional sex workers. Because of this, the principles and methods of Motivational Interviewing (MI), a prominent "evidence-based" technique in the treatment of substance abuse and dependence, are referenced less frequently in sex addiction treatment circles and literature.

Motivational Interviewing, 12-Step Programs, and Initial Assessment

MI methods eschew therapists' use of counter-statements designed to confront patients or interpret their resistance. MI also avoids educative pronouncements. Instead, MI practitioners employ empathetic statements that mirror patients' extant positions, "rolling with resistance" rather than countering it (Miller & Rollnick, 2002). Giudice and Kutinsky (2007) presented cases in which MI techniques were applied to individuals presenting with a history of sexually compulsive behaviors. They used these case illustrations to proclaim the efficacy of the approach and speculate that a wider use of MI with respect to sex addiction was indicated. Are these techniques employed less in sex addiction treatment because they are less effective? Are some addictions deemed more conducive to a nondirective approach than others? Probably not. However, if MI has found less traction in sex addiction than in chemical dependency, it's likely not because of abstinence-proselytizing 12-step sponsors, or the demands of the would-be addict. Instead, we speculate that ambivalent motivation may be less tolerated when a relational system, rather than an individual, is the presenting unit of treatment. How might directive sex addiction therapists reconcile the principles of MI with honesty agreements and disclosure exercises in the context of shameful exposure and sexual betrayal? And how do you "roll with resistance" while pressuring someone to take a polygraph exam? As for continued acting out, when the unit (a couple) presents for treatment, the prospect of relapse, especially a direct-contact episode of sexual acting out, is so unacceptable it scarcely bears thinking about.

It seems ironic that a popular 12-step program related to sex addiction—Sex Addicts Anonymous (SAA)—actually does not recommend abstinence per se as a standard by which a person's recovery is measured. In this way, SAA differs from its parent fellowships, Alcoholics Anonymous (AA) and Narcotics Anonymous (NA). Because sex is not deemed intrinsically poisonous to the body and mind of afflicted persons, SAA doesn't suppose that abstinence from sex is the goal of recovery. It doesn't seek to render people asexual. Instead, it recommends a guideline system known as the three circles that serve to direct a person's thinking about their sexuality to evoke a plan that will fit their value system. It is an implicitly individualized model, not one that caters to an impacted system. If it did, then the notable 9th step of a 12-step program, in which recovering addicts are meant to make amends to impacted others, would likely get bumped to a higher step.

Anyway, regarding the three circles of SAA: Inner circle behavior is the set of behaviors that a person most wishes to avoid, such as porn use or sex outside of a committed relationship. The middle circle, or "slippery" territory, represents behaviors that may lead a person to their inner circle, sometimes called a "bottom line." Examples of middle circle behaviors include patterns of browsing online images that may not be pornographic but are intriguing; and patterns of flirting or excessive fantasy, with or without masturbation. Nonsexual behaviors such as isolating or avoiding fellowship might also be considered middle circle activity, as they are not conducive to a conscious-seeking recovery lifestyle. The third, or outer circle of SAA, less understood because it receives less attention, pertains to healthy, recovery-seeking activities, which may be—but aren't necessarily—nonsexual. The outer circle is both a derivative concept (sublimation) and shorthand for unmet needs. Such needs may be non-specific but might include wholesome hobbies and, especially in the context of men's-only or women's-only groups, same-sex comradeship. Most importantly, this outer circle pertains to activities and thoughts that do not induce excessive guilt and shame, suggesting that they needn't be kept secret.

When a couple presents in the aftermath of discovery, seeking treatment for the acting out behavior, it's best to meet with the acting out party first, so that person can be screened for what he'd done, how often and for how long he'd done it, and then what he's willing to share in therapy or with a prospective support group. "What about *her?*" the would-be patient may ask, glancing at the wall separating the office from a waiting area where she waits, hoping or expecting to take part in the process—or not.

It might be tempting to think of their experiences as separate and treat one person individually or via a group process, referring the other partner to someone else. However, it is neither possible nor wise to attempt this separation completely. At the very least, an assessment of systemic intent is called for. The acting out partner can't proceed easily without considering his nonacting out partner, and vice versa. So, the clinician must endure the uneasy tension on both sides, perhaps explaining to each partner that, while their treatment may not be coordinated explicitly, they will still be asked to *think* about the other's experience. A couple may be disgruntled or even shocked to find their clinicians warning against too much talking (to each other) at first. Or, some couples may be relieved by this proscription, thinking they'd rather not speak to each other at all.

The therapeutic intent is to build on a foundation by applying (but not relying on) assessment tools such as the Sex Addiction Assessment (SAST) or the Hypersexual Behavior (HB-19) questionnaire (two of the less dense tools available). Regardless of what such assessments reveal, we refrain from using the word addict, wary of the syllogism that often accompanies that term: if X is an addict, then theoretical insight Y applies. Formulaic solutions often follow. Operating on the belief that couples beset with infidelity or other sexual problems have suffered in isolation, we point them in the direction of support groups, aimed separately at men and women. Such groups provide emotional succor and a respite from hostile exchanges and judgment. Would-be sex addicts tend to be more receptive, thinking they have little choice but to accept an "expert" directive, as the stage of being indignant in response to accusations is over—discovery put an end to that. Impacted partners may be more confused, asking why they need support. What do they need to talk about?

While some men presenting for sex addiction treatment are angry, disdainful of mental health interventions, or open to consultation but not the stacked deck of presumptuous care, the majority of men in this context seem docile, escapist, and guilt-ridden. They are indentured by their sins, willing to make some concessions and cooperate. They are not confused about what they do, when and how often they do it, or even why they do it in a superficial sense. They are confused about the underlying reasons for their behavior: the secondary, deeper purposes of their destructive acts; their disappearances from love and self. How terrible is it to want to stop doing something—to promise not to do it to yourself, even—only to keep doing that thing?

And the betrayed partners are not all angry, panic-stricken, or dismissive women. Though belatedly introduced to unpleasant truths, they are typically dug into the fabric of their lives, with their partners inhabiting the center. They may expect monogamy, but not necessarily monogamist thought. Financial dependence is often a factor that deters impulsive decisions to separate from acting out men and from their own humiliation. At the same time, they may feel that not leaving is subject to judgment, imagining the cold, knowing glances of other, less financially dependent women. The needs of children are also taken into account. There is a bias toward stability and the value of presenting a united parental front, which among other things means not destroying the good image of the father. Then there's the sticky matter of love. Most of the women we've observed in these scenarios still love the men who have let them down. Whatever the treatment process implies as to their role in marital problems, that not-so-easily discarded bond may be the reason they stick around.

Patients relax if they find their treating professionals friendly, casual, and not judging them for porn habits, prostitution-seeking, or affairs. As they share the details of their misdeeds and the impact on their partners, they might wonder about their therapists, our habits. After all, isn't much of their behavior normal—for men, they mean? Just how big is the porn industry, anyway? Isn't casual sex just a few clicks or swipes away on websites that cater to a variety of tastes? And what about prostitution? The massage establishments that front brothels are clearly aimed at a male clientele, and in some cities seem more plentiful than convenience stores. The men who sit with us after having spent years plus thousands of dollars frequenting such places live in the same world that their therapists live in. We share roughly the same temptations, observe the same beauteous physicality of women, and experience similar pressures to act on sexual urges within ourselves more or less constantly (age factors notwithstanding). A patient may at least wonder if their therapist knows what it's like to ache for sex, or to live with a woman whose libido doesn't measure up, or to love one woman but find countless others attractive.

Therapists, especially male therapists, inhabit a special position in this corner of mental health treatment. We're meant to coach behavioral strategies from the perspective of men, helping patients to restore moral rectitude and take responsibility in a behavioral sense, in keeping with some traditional standard that men are meant to echo to one another. We represent sexual probity even if we don't present ourselves that way. In this way, we are unlike 12-step sponsors, who are weathervanes in their sexual recovery. Sponsors are prone to relapses that they are ethically bound to share with peers, including the sponsees who they guide. For the shadow consumer that is womankind, male therapists serve as mind mechanics and relationship guides. We're part of a redeemer class of males, tasked with shepherding our remedial brethren into a more intuitive, right-brain way of being.

Money, Time, and Shame: Three Indices of Assessment

Alongside an inventory of acting out behaviors, the grounding of structure and interventionist plans, and a review of the plainer consequences of discovery, a clinician and patient, working together within a psychodynamic framework, might explore some of the other less talked about aspects of porn use and transactional sex, including money, time, and shame. For many patients entering treatment, money and time have governed the onset and progression of their problem behaviors. Money, of course, dictates whether prostitutes can be employed, how frequently they can be visited, the quality of the provider, and the services rendered. Asking about money spent on prostitution is a standard question in an assessment protocol, intended to uncover the scale of activity.

> One patient reported that he'd spent $10,000 during a discrete decadent phase. Assuming he was estimating an aggregate total from an acting out pattern, I naively asked him to define the period in which he'd spent that much money. "One night," he replied, seeming a bit thrown by the question. He wasn't boasting. Money was simply no object. Fantasies were.

Time is another significant factor. Time and space are both necessary for acting out to occur without detection. There must be gaps in schedules, time not accounted for. If time is short, then acting out must be as well. Hence the need for "quickies," which can include anonymous partners or "hook-ups" through websites aimed at those with little desire for a relationship as that concept is conventionally defined.

Time limits compete with ego ideals concerning porn. Recognizing that time is a commodity, producers of porn have effected ingenious developments over the last generation or so. In the last 30 to 40 years, porn has moved from sordid downtown theaters to the videotape, to the computer, and finally to the smartphone, with each transition rendering it more accessible, more private, and—perhaps above all—more time-efficient. Porn can now be used during a homework break or, with a sly look over the shoulder, after a stressful work email has been sent. Porn can be used in a bathroom stall, as long as the search history is thoroughly "wiped" after use. Sex addiction specialists ask about preferences and tastes because there are genres: Hub this and hub that. On the other end of the time scale, porn can consume great chunks of time on a day off, as users compulsively search for that perfect image, a certain angle, a few magical seconds of a clip, or a specific look in a "hot" person's eye when browsing dating or "hook-up" sites. For many, porn and dating bleed together in a sort of digital cross-pollination. Such perfection-seeking is a brain freeze, a death instinct march. Time and feeling may fly by unnoticed until eyelids flicker and a quick glance catches a digital clock read-out, prompting disbelief or self-disgust to settle in and increase fatigue. The men we typically listen to aren't proud of the time they've spent over a lifetime or during any given episode of chasing women or looking at porn. Despite the calamitous discoveries that precipitate treatment, many seem far more disturbed by this consequence of lost time than by any notion of betrayal to a loving partner, which says something about time's material and psychic value.

Porn generates both shame and guilt for several reasons. For some, porn use accompanies masturbation, an equally shameful habit for some. It is potential wasted sex outside of marriage or relationship, and some can't bear to think about it, much less talk about it. Once upon a time, masturbation was grounds for castration and was seen as depriving the body of essential fluids contained in semen. But the fear that accompanies shame extends beyond morality to low self-esteem and feelings of inadequacy. The implication of the voyeuristic act, after all, is that sex doesn't exist in the self or isn't vital enough, so the habitual porn user must find sex in others. These men sometimes graduate or progress to exhibitionism or cross-dressing because they envy others, especially women, who seem confident to manifest their sexuality by displaying their bodies, preening, posing, and *performing*. From an aesthete's point of view, sex exists legitimately in fashion and in art. So, in one respect porn is merely bad art, art that isn't missed when it's gone, making the craving for it a strangely muted outcry. Thoughts of porn stir sexual desire, but the user rarely feels sexy. Passion is absent. So, the repeated association of images with stimulation, which becomes more predictable and routinized with each successive episode, may even lead to impotence. This unintended consequence may be a sign that the porn user's sexuality has become ineffectually linked to a false experience of sex. When a "failure to perform" occurs, the resultant shame and isolation, replete with irritable mutterings, glazed expressions, and shifty apologies, compounds the shame associated with porn and a deeper shame about which the afflicted person may be quite unaware.

Being unaware of shame is an experience that everyone should have at least once. Not blissfully unaware, perhaps, but everyone deserves a moment of relative ease, of anodyne sexuality, before there is trouble. For some people, the first forbidden behavior may have been like their first taste of alcohol, a whiff of a cigarette, or the use of some other illicit substance. It brings to mind a time when sexuality was a positive happening and elicits fond recognition of events such as a stolen kiss, a bravura dance move; flowers delivered before an intended deflowering. They recall the high, plus a sense of mischief—a childhood memory of doing something naughty and then getting away with it. It seems that mischief is one of adulthood's forgotten needs, a Winnicottian experience of self via play (Winnicott, 1971). Mischief conjures the delight that you feel when you break the rules, don't wait your turn, or hide under the dining room table and from adults. Patients often dreamily recall earlier, less damaging episodes: stealing time away from work, school, or some onerous family obligation, only to return poker-faced to polite society, acting as nothing has happened. We love the experience of being unwitnessed, the feeling of freedom. These first sexual indiscretions were part rite of passage and part adventure, not harbingers of addiction and relationship pain. They were coming-of-age moments long before they were albatrosses, scarlet letters, or secrets that did harm.

Female Sex and Love Addiction: The Under-Researched and Under-Treated

And what about the mischief of girls? The treatment of female sexual addiction is framed differently than that of male sex addicts, with arguments that obscure today's fraught ethics with hoary gender bias pronouncements. In an overview of female sex and love addiction (FSLA) treatment, Ferree (2012) contrasted treatment of women with the treatment of men by outlining distinctive elements of the female sex addict profile.

First, the sexual activity of FSLAs incurs some harsher consequences that, if repetitive, place women at greater risk for cervical cancer, unwanted pregnancies, or date rape victimization. Also, women tend to face lesser legal consequences for comparable sexual offenses (like exhibitionism), but they are more likely to be arrested for practicing prostitution than men are as consumers. Beyond that, the observations of FSLAs by practitioners and authors are largely anecdotal and speculative, but seem more credulous: They indicate that women report romance-oriented problems, like excessive flirting, pursuing relationships with married or otherwise unavailable men, or trading sex for drugs. The keyword here is *report*. Aren't they getting in trouble, being caught by angry partners or a sex-policing, stigmatizing society? Commentators across media assert that FSLA is under-researched and under-treated, implying that women have been deprived of care, such as the presumed benefits of sex addiction labeling. Authors like Ferree (2012) or Weiss (2013) assert that female sex addicts view their behaviors in terms of relationships.[5] Like men, they disregard sexual boundaries, but they do so with consensual partners, hence the relative absence of terms like "objectification," "harassment," or "misconduct" from the lexicon that confronts FSLA behavior.

Next, Ferree (2012) argued that women are deterred from seeking treatment because they are subject to especially shaming terms like "slut," "whore," or "nymphomaniac." (The masculine-inflected terms "creep," "pervert," or "pig" are relative endearments, we infer.) This argument presupposes that candidates for treatment volunteer for care rather than being mandated by a court or an angry spouse. The stigmatizing of women would be moot if

5. This assertion appears to parallel a shift in psychoanalysis: in relational or feminist psychoanalysis, a psyche is formed via internalizations. Being in a relationship is deemed a primary need (Bowlby, 1960; Winnicott, 1971). This contrasts with the theories of Freud (1905) and Klein (1928, 1935) in which relationships are secondary and are used to satisfy a drive. The distinction is important and it's fascinating that observations of male sex addicts tend to echo the classical theories, while insights about women conspicuously reflect the newer relational lens.

these women had broken the law or gaslighted their partners, who might then reach out to treatment centers, expecting rigorous intervention and demanding change. If this doesn't happen so much, the reasons haven't really been studied, but that doesn't halt the narrative-building. The paradoxical/inverted logic goes something like this: men's promiscuity or sexual compulsivity is more socially acceptable than the corresponding behavior of women, so society focuses on changing the behavior of . . . men? Something's not right with this picture. Yes, men are considered "studs" for being promiscuous. However, they're not exactly lauded for binging on porn or for seeking prostitutes, and it's the ubiquity of these outlets that is most implicated in current sex addiction theories, not a revolution in affair-seeking behavior. With shame-mitigating purpose, many therapists opine that women are more "relational." This reflects a broader belief that women are more empathetic, which is based on studies indicating that women sense the stress of children more readily than men or those conducted with female-only samples, or inconclusive studies that show slightly more responsiveness to nonverbal cues in communication in women than in men.

These stereotypes indicate that women are motivated by love, not sex as a purely physical act or an act of play. The related assertion that "women are nurturers by nature" implies that men are less nurturing. The analogous masculine chestnut, "men are problem-solvers," likewise implies that women are deficient in this area. Here's a less partisan view: problem-solving, whether stereotypically male or not, is a version of nurturing, so comparisons of nurturing styles ultimately reflect bias, or incomplete or culture-bound assumptions. Anyway, the relational qualifier is intended to connote a warmer, more intimate, and humanizing purpose for an FSLA's acting out behaviors, which is surely unfair to all the male love addicts who crave soul connections and find them with women named Raven or Destiny. This FSLA profile is based on anecdotal evidence or extrapolated from a broader conceptualization of women's sexuality to explain behaviors that contain power-seeking or misandrist elements:

- Acting out born of abusive ties with fathers (Opitz et al., 2009).
- Teasing behaviors like sexting or stalking (Sharon-Perez, 2009; Sussman, 2010, as cited in Ferree, 2012).

Such findings reveal tautological attitudes that engender sympathies for FSLAs, making them seem a bit like an endangered yet protected species. So, men's porn use and other problem sexual behaviors objectify women. Women's porn use and other problem sexual behaviors objectify women. This is a circular narrative: the premise remains fixed regardless of the variables. Therefore, FSLAs are treated as victims of social stigma, past or present physical abuse, or generalized social disadvantage. The following axiom is widely accepted by treatment providers: Women do not exploit or objectify; instead, they are exploited and objectified, either by men or by their internalization of social disregard.

Sex Addiction, Personality, and Attachment Disorder

In programs that treat sex addiction, patients are subject not only to assessments of their sex addiction, but to personality profiles as well. Despite the common belief among professionals that personality disorder diagnoses should be deferred while sobriety is pursued (allowing for personality to stabilize), patients in short-term sex addiction treatment programs are often subject to personality testing and may be discharged after just a few weeks with labels or diagnoses such as sex addict or Narcissistic Personality Disorder, with little understanding of the meaning of those terms. Yeomans et al. (1993), Linehan et al. (2007), and Sansone et al. (2011) observed comorbidity of high-risk sexual behaviors in women with Borderline Personality Disorder. Meares (2012) writes as if Borderline Personality and dissociative disorders (such as PTSD, an anxiety disorder with dissociative features) are more or less synonymous terms. This echoes findings such as those by Zanarini and colleagues, whose study of 358 Borderline patients indicated that 91% of subjects had reported childhood abuse (Zanarini et al., 1997). As for Narcissistic Personality Disorder, the assignment of that diagnosis to sex addicts is largely heuristic and appears to reflect social disapproval of affairs, prostitution-seeking, or porn use rather than research, clinical observation, or even a fair cross-section of social values. Narcissism is inferred with respect to prostitution and porn use because the behavior seems egoistic, with little concern by the consumer for the welfare or pleasure of the desired objects. Concerning infidelity, observers may infer that admiration-seeking, while more personal than the objectifying motives linked to porn and prostitution, also reflects a miscreant, narcissistic aim.

From a psychoanalytic perspective, the elucidation of Borderline Personality Disorder or Narcissistic Personality Disorder is a prodigious task. However, for the purposes of treatment, it might be a gratuitous rabbit hole. Reid et al. (2013) suggest that research linking personality disorders with sexual acting out behaviors is inconclusive, indicating that it is confounded by limited sample size, questionable subject recruitment methods, and varying definitions of sex addiction. What about varying notions of personality? Like the offhand notion that women are more hard-wired for relationship-seeking than men, the link between narcissism and sex addiction, for example, is not a standardized professional opinion. It is simply what a lot of people think, so the idea is an easy sell to consumers.

In modern psychology's first major foray into the subject, Freud (1914a, 1917) explored narcissism as a state of infantile existence. Echoing the classic Greek myth from which the condition is derived, and filtering through the later Copernican revolution in cosmology, Freud posited that narcissism is first an auto-erotic state, diminished but not fully renounced when invested in another. At later stages of development, individuals set up an ideal of who they want to be, a proto-superego in Freud's early thinking. This idea was later echoed by self psychologists, most notably Kohut (1971), as a development of healthy separateness. Alternatively, a version of Narcissistic Personality Disorder generates perfection-seeking and overvaluation of ideals, resulting in a regressive, melancholic withdrawal from objects (caregivers or others) that is underlined by moralistic—if secret—self-reproaches and engulfment within another. Masterson (1981) built on this idea, plus the later object relations theory of Klein (1928, 1935, 1946) and the developmental theory of Mahler (1975), asserting that narcissistic disorders proceed from excessive gratification within stages of toddlerhood:

> The fantasy persists that the world is his oyster and revolves about him. In order to protect this illusion, he must seal off by avoidance, denial and devaluation those perceptions of reality that do not fit or resonate with this narcissistic, grandiose self-projection. (Masterson, 1981, p. 13)

The extrapolated conception of narcissism, which involves both hypersexualization of and de-cathecting from objects, includes lack of empathy for and exploitation of others. It casts excessive pleasure-seeking as an act of domineering arrogance, echoing an old belief that the sun revolves around the earth, not the reverse. The diagnostic view ignores that narcissism is often perceived as charming. Also, from a polyamorous or feminist perspective, marriage constitutes possession, especially possession of women, so jealous love or exclusivity might also be deemed narcissistic love. For sex addiction, a term that implies non-monogamous sex, perceptions of narcissism betray value judgments that vary depending upon worldviews. Therefore, despite its importance as a phenomenon of loss, narcissism has become one of the most weaponized terms in modern psychology—a word used to demarcate who does and who does not merit drawing attention to themselves.

And what of other pathological personality presentations, like Schizoid Personality Disorder? If someone presenting for treatment appears to exhibit porn use only, relates more to machines (computers) than to other human beings, eschews direct contact in their sexual acting out, and demonstrates safety-seeking (rather than risk-taking) behaviors across relational contexts, a diagnosis of Schizoid Personality Disorder might be considered. As profiled by several object relations theorists (Fairbairn, 1944; Guntrip, 1969; Masterson & Klein, 1995; Ogden, 1989), a Schizoid pattern is primarily related to distancing, not grandiosity, admiration, or intimacy-seeking. A Schizoid may desire connection with others, but does so thinly to avoid loss of autonomy, settling for invisibility (in place of praise) and fearing exploitation (though colluding with it passively via porn use). The risk of being caught deters affairs. When asked why he *didn't* progress from porn addiction to prostitute or affair-seeking behavior, one patient gave a Schizoid-like response, saying that he dreaded persecution, adding that he'd never want to have sex with a woman who disliked him, because she might do him harm. Dread is important because it signifies the imminence of negative outcomes, not just the possibility. Fear can be thought about. Dread stifles action and thought. Contingencies appear to matter less to narcissistic personalities. For them, gambling is a stimulant. Unfortunately, there's a paucity of literature on comorbidity of sex addiction and Schizoid functioning. It's as if an *a priori* belief permeates mental health systems: Narcissism is the personality type comorbid with hypersexual behaviors and addictions in general, with Borderline Personality Disorder the preferred diagnosis for women. This may be addiction doctrine, but it doesn't help clinicians observe the nuances of motivation among patients presenting for treatment.

Many patients enter therapy with vague descriptions of insecure attachment styles that they import from previous therapeutic episodes. Unsurprisingly, sex addiction treatment programs have drawn on attachment theory to explain the origin of patients' affect dysregulation. Carnes (1991) reported that 78% of sex addicts come from rigidly disengaged families. More recently, Zitzman and Butler (2009) opined that pornography reinforces a nonintimate, nonrelational sexual experience. Attachment theory holds that an infant's attachment to a caregiver is internalized as a working model of attachment, which in turn influences proximity-seeking behavior (Bowlby, 1960). Further, Strange Situation studies devised by Ainsworth et al. (1978) and Main and Solomon (1986) led to attachment categorizations that correlate with "state of mind" or Adult Attachment Inventory classifications:

- Secure attachment engenders fluidity in narrative-building and capacities for self-reflection and access to memory.
- An avoidant type features marked tendencies toward emotional distancing.
- An ambivalent or resistant attachment style is exhibited in those who seem uncertain in relationships and can be clinging and demanding but also distancing.
- Disorganized attachment style manifests as dissociative habits, collapsing or freezing in stressful situations.

Until recently, it was thought that sexual dimorphism did not pertain to attachment disorders, but Schore (2016) assembled research suggesting that stress-regulating circuits of the male brain mature more slowly. Male newborns maintain eye contact less, fuss and cry more, and react to stressful situations with higher cortisol levels resulting from epigenetic factors (both prenatal and postnatal) such as higher levels of testosterone. Regarding the impact of mothers, Bertrand and Pan (2013) documented that boys raised in single-mother homes show twice the rate of behavioral problems compared to children from two-parent homes, and that single mothers spend less time with male infants than with female infants.

However, boys may "catch up" in terms of social and emotional development by adulthood, as roughly equal percentages (48% of males and 50% of females) are reported as securely attached on Adult Attachment Interviews (Schore, 2016). Lastly, Siegel (1999) cautioned that insecure attachment is not equivalent to personality disorder, PTSD, or an "addictive" personality, but rather "creates a risk of later psychological and social dysfunction" (Siegel, 1999, p. 84).

Splitting, "Excuses," and Keys to Therapy

In our offices, we often see patients who have emerged from short-term sex addiction treatment programs armed with a catalog of vocabulary derived from OR theory or attachment theory. However, this vocabulary is usually not credited to either framework, but to the metaphors of computer programming, as in "you were programmed to . . ." Consumers read books or articles that feature recommendations like "find someone who understands sex addiction," which typically means those who subscribe to the model founded by Patrick Carnes. Such recommendations imply that practitioners who don't readily assign the term sex addiction to their patients don't understand the condition and are therefore unfit to provide care. The labels and jargon imparted to patients, watered down from theoretical antecedents to be inclusive, become the clothing that shapes an aftercare process. This process is meant to evolve and lead to deepening self-awareness. But long after the short-term programs have ceased, the notions from early interventions often remain, fossilizing roles like perpetrator and victim against the supposition that time and therapy might provide nuanced interpretations. The problem of overidentification and labeling is illustrated in the following example:

> A sexually acting out man bemoans his last slip and revisits with incredulity the consequences of his continuing habits. Breaking out a paper containing his reflections (his "homework"), he details a chronology of events with seeming accuracy and is eloquent in his contrition but lacks insight. Instead, he falls back on terminology that has organized and contained his behavior, but not expanded his awareness. When asked why he did what he did in the moment or moments of so-called triggering, he shrugs and summarizes, saying "because that's what I am . . . an addict."

Obfuscations like this one are among the reasons why some regard 12-step programs as cults, and consider the term sex addiction an excuse. Setting aside the issue of medical legitimacy, it's not that "addict" identifications are inappropriate, but they are limiting. It's not that terms like "victim" or "perpetrator" are wholly wrong, but they can be either inflammatory or dull; they reignite primitive defenses and split reality into binary conditions, recalling Klein's (1928, 1946) description of infantile psychic processes. Addiction rhetoric can foster bland introspection on dense, confusing relationships. Instead of beginning a thought process, some circumscribe it, packaging it neatly so that they can move on quickly, in keeping with economic paradigms that drive the industrious work ethic prized by a materialistic society.

Also, it's not that sex addiction excuses problem sexual behavior. It's that using the term to punctuate insight excuses not thinking more fully about the problem. In the sustained treatment of would-be sex addicts and their partners, the longer-term aim is to focus on the internal process of elusive split-off feeling states, not just behaviors, which are the externalization of thought. Melanie Klein originally defined splitting as a primitive but necessary defense; it keeps good and bad separate to protect the self as well as a loved caregiver. In later development, splitting represents the struggle to hold feelings of good and bad about self and others simultaneously. If healthy, or whole, we hold pleasure and pain, lust and love together in our minds rather than expelling or compartmentalizing these feelings to avoid pain. Splitting results in alternating states of idealization and devaluation, making integration, or feeling whole, difficult.

As clinicians, we tend to perceive splitting when we are being devalued, especially when complaints reach others' ears. Clinical managers working as team leads in treatment agencies tend to give the concept of splitting a plainer systemic meaning than the one provided by object relations theory. Eschewing the intrapsychic, they describe splitting as a behavior in which patients attempt to play one therapist against another, like a manipulative child interacting with their parents through reenactments, telling lies, and presenting different faces to different people.

In the effort to defeat splitting as it is behaviorally defined, treatment teams might share numerous "secrets" of their clients, not just to thwart acting out sexual behaviors or acts that merit crisis intervention, but to counter a variety of thoughts that may be undermining desired outcomes. The confidentiality implications of professional collaboration (especially concerning so-called slips in acting out behavior) are covered more fully in the illustration of Kevork and Shannon in Chapter 6. However, this subject impacts all formats of therapy, not just couples work. If, as a therapist, you are sitting with someone who flatters you, devalues you by pointing out the more effective method of another therapist, or else disturbs your understanding with representations of others' statements, it's not your job to summon all pertinent witnesses, as in some manner of village hearing. It's not the job of a colleague to rebuke a patient on your behalf, or the job of a consultant spouse or parent to confirm or dispel your patient's assertions. It is your job to acknowledge wrongdoing when appropriate but maintain your competency. It is your job to maintain your position with patients who may fire you for not assuming a desired and predicted role. It is important to take feedback with a grain of salt and to be neutral yet human. It's important that patients experience you as good and bad yet available and un-destroyed by primitive defenses such as splitting.

When working within a psychodynamic framework with someone who presents as a sex addict or with problem sexual behaviors, it's important to distinguish between behavioral and intrapsychic understandings of splitting defenses. A psychodynamic clinician's bias is to help understand problems, not co-manage them, and it may be necessary to pivot quickly when presented with a challenge like the following:

> Six months after a patient presenting as a sex addict with a betrayed partner has entered individual therapy with you, he and his partner have entered into couples therapy with a systems-oriented practitioner. The patient has authorized the couple's therapist to collaborate with you. According to protocols defined by other approaches, there are boundaries regarding what to tell children and extended family; ground rules regarding the living situation to be worked out; and a full-disclosure exercise to be coordinated. The couple's therapist calls and asks cloaked questions like "the partner just wants to know if he's working on his narcissism." In effect, such questions ask you to reveal disclosed information from an individual session that bypasses or might even contradict what may have been said in a couple's session.

Suddenly, you are more of an informant than an analytically informed therapist, and no one involved will think that this renders psychotherapy a performance except you. At this point, your patient's understanding of the process is crucial, because the popularity of the systemic approach is undeniable. If your patient has a long-term commitment to working on his self and to disclosing confidential material that protects the treatment, a psychodynamic framework may prevail, minimizing collateral communications. Coordinating interventions for the system's benefit is based (incorrectly) on a belief that individual therapists have obligations to meet the non-emergency needs of a patient's spouse. However, if it's all about happy other or happy self or the presumed virtues of teamwork (having everyone "on the same page"), a deepening process may be compromised, perhaps irreparably.

Practitioners inclined toward a psychodynamic approach, familiar with attachment theory, OR theory, and advances in neurobiology, might observe splitting and projections (those unconscious assumptions that people direct at one another). Because the concept of complex trauma sometimes conflates sexual betrayals and personality disorder, be careful that labels like victim (or its euphemistic synonym, survivor) do not become thought-arresting identifications. If the hyper-aroused or dissociative responses of partners seem to predate exposure of the designated sex addict, practitioners needn't accept a partner's inference that trauma only began at disclosure, even if they don't contest this supposition in early treatment. More explicitly, if observing trauma-based hyperarousal and hypervigilance, clinicians needn't indulge fear-based partner beliefs, expressed via questions like "will he molest my children?" These represent prejudices about sex addicts that are not substantiated by research (Seto et al., 2011). Clinicians should be mindful of transference and countertransference, and of primitive defenses like splitting and projective identification (the inducement of split-off feelings in another). They should manifest patience in the treatment of complex dynamics, be aware of their own capacities for dissociation, and not provide rote solutions simply because familiar tools are demanded by anxious consumers.

To summarize, we propose in-depth, psychodynamic, thought- and feeling-provoking therapy for a self-identified or would-be sex addict that entails the following:

- Developing an understanding of unrecognized needs obscured by sexual preoccupation.
- Understanding feeling states that underlay acting out, splitting, intellectualizing defenses, and internalizing object relations.
- Understanding the experiences of a nonacting out partner and any fantasy objects.
- Discussing fantasies deemed objectionable by polite society.
- Contemplating addiction as repetitive, and distancing it from the self.
- Understanding transference responses: a reexperiencing of emotional relationships with origins in earliest object-attachments.
- Attending to actual and potential enactments in the therapeutic relationship.

It's not easy to engage in real discussion about sex, let alone deviant or supposedly objectionable sex. Other than death, sex is *the* most difficult subject, and it's hardly made easier in the context of a mental or behavioral disorder. Absent comic distraction, a man presenting for sex addiction treatment scrambles to find words to describe sensitive material, or the correct rhetoric to express sober regret for past behavior and a determination to change. If excited or possibly relieved to find the chance to speak freely, an open-minded and talkative patient might embark on a discussion of his psychology, thinking that there is much to learn. Perhaps eager to be heard with genuine interest and compassion, such a patient might share stories, painted with details that sound and feel different or somehow better when spoken aloud. He might describe the typical scene, time of day, and conditions, such as isolation, that enable his escapism, or what happens in his mind when he feels restless, how he is activated to fantasize, and how memories of his experience regularly taunt him. Conscious of being free but not lonely or fearful of missing out (FOMO, millennials tell us), he'll dimly consider what's missing from his habitual pleasure. He might observe the beauty of perfection, or the easy, carefree scenarios that make sex possible for some, and indulge vicariously. But the women he obsesses over aren't made real in daylight, and the scenarios suggesting freedom are neither likely nor satisfying, ultimately.

In particular, two attitudes tend to block thoughtful discussion of sex addiction: excuses and scapegoating. One is that sex addiction, as an assessment or diagnostic term, is an excuse contrived by philanderers, perverts, and their apologists to give psychiatric meaning to immoral behavior and leverage social clemency. For some, the sex addiction label is proof that treatment privileges acting out men, not their partners. The "excuse" complaint implies that impacted partners are necessarily less incentivized to accept the addiction label and presumes that self-identified addicts deflect rather than absorb blame for relationship problems. Well, it does seem opportunistic when a high-profile celebrity or politician admits himself to sex addiction treatment soon after sexual misconduct has come to light. Such high-profile cases also skew the public perception of sex addiction concerning social class. Expensive, short-term residential treatment programs cater to those whose behaviors have been extravagant, involving scores of partners, heavy expenditures on acting out, affairs, or prostitution-seeking rather than porn. At the same time, there is no special sympathy afforded sex addicts simply because they self-diagnose. For the less celebrated and the less affluent, discovery of a sexual acting out pattern merits intervention, delivered in a manner that preserves dignity. However, a mental health intervention is not mutually exclusive of potentially punitive legal or personal decisions. The fact that someone is in sex addiction treatment does not preclude a divorce action or a decision to separate by a nonacting out partner. It also does not mitigate a criminal sentence in the event of a sexual offense, although in such cases, mandated referrals to treatment might supplement sentences. It is not a clinician's job to convince a betrayed spouse to remain committed to a habitually sexually acting out person any more than it is to support or effect the exile of the misbehaving figure.

The offhand rejection of addiction as a psychological phenomenon also blocks thinking, substituting a moralizing dimension that tends to thwart further discussion. Those who express the "excuse" view tend to not accept that some are more vulnerable to anxious or depressive states than others. They reject the notion that some people have less capacity for impulse control, executive decision-making, or frustration tolerance. Or, if such deficits are acknowledged, they think it the responsibility of the afflicted party to contend with their conditions, to *deal with them*. Such protestations may seem correct, but they are also facile and may be delivered harshly, according to self-identified addicts or those in 12-step circles.

However, this prejudice isn't as toxic as the addiction-as-scapegoat argument, which can hinder the therapeutic process even more. At its worst, it's a habit of another kind: a trump card in a dispute that serves as a climactic, circular insight. "All roads lead to my acting out," a patient may complain, referring to the futility of discussion with a betrayed spouse. In ongoing fights, ostensibly nonsexual behaviors are attributed to psychological or spiritual dimensions of a multi-layered addiction. If the patient is inattentive in a private discussion, it is because he is daydreaming—a dissociative symptom of his addiction. If he forgets to attend to an important familial or domestic task, this too is linked to his addictive pattern. If he bristles at his partner's suspicions, asks for sex when his wife isn't interested, or doesn't "validate" his wife's steadfast belief that he'd ogled the waitress at a restaurant on their so-called date night, he is manifesting aspects of his addiction: being in denial, lying, and lacking empathy by not owning the accusations leveled at him. In such exchanges, addiction becomes an umbrella term, comprised of manifold comorbidities.

The would-be sex addict might despair at this point, thinking that normative disputes will always be tilted in the direction of his partner's biases. He thinks that nothing can ever be truly discussed because his condition—his sentence, so to speak—is the meaning underlying all of his problems. He becomes passive and speaks resignedly, employing tautologies like "it is what it is." This is perhaps an exaggerated depiction of those partners who have learned—or decided, without apology—that their partner's addiction is the defining problem impacting the couple.

For these impacted partners, the addiction-as-scapegoat position replaces the previous gaslighting phenomenon in which the nonacting out person's paranoia, controlling tendencies, careless accusations, overly critical nature, and overall "craziness" were the previous narratives of a longstanding impasse. In such cases, discovery revealed more than a pattern of acting out and the breakdown of the addict's denial system. It also marked a shift in the dynamics of the relationship, a cataclysmic forfeiture of power, from the viewpoint of the fallen other. Now the accusations, persistent questions, cell phone monitoring, search history inventories, and general distrust become sanctioned or witnessed by a guardrail of support if the partner shares her concerns with others. The discovered, acting out partner is more or less compelled to yield power if he wants to stay in the relationship, and might even sign a document agreeing to his partner's terms, like a defeated army signing an armistice. The capacity to grow via this loss (rather than fight it) often marks the difference between relationships that last and those that don't.

CASE ILLUSTRATION: NOT THINKING (MR. A)

Not thinking before acting: this epitomizes the addict, it seems. This is a stereotype, and a laconic view of addiction, but one shared by psychoanalysis, perhaps. The addict plots, devises, and anticipates obstacles, but does not reflect, making him unable to foresee variable outcomes of a decision. Consequences! The addict does not foresee consequences, which later becomes the overriding focus of the concerned family, and the addiction specialists who will treat him. He does not think about past bad decisions, as they stir painful memories: "It's best not to *dwell* on them." He further struggles to observe either his own feelings and inner needs or those of others, and this problem pervades day-to-day matters. At times psychotic, he may lack the capacity to tolerate frustration, be unable to employ the reality principle, and will treat thought itself as a bad object, "indistinguishable from a thing-in-itself, fit only for evacuation" (Bion, 1962, p. 307). Still, direct discussion about feelings might cause twitches of cognitive dissonance. The addict accepts that his inability to notice feelings is a problem. At the same time, he might think it best to avoid focusing on dysphoric feelings by taking his mind off them with, well . . . you know. At some point he may acknowledge this contradiction, or at least observe that this modus operandi isn't working. Healthy alternative behaviors, like reflective thought, *dwelling*, aren't being chosen. Why? The person feels discomfort, but instead of thinking about the feeling, he blocks thought, which in turn means that informed choice of action is also blocked.

> Mr. A is a self-described sex addict who entered therapy proclaiming deep guilt and a determination to change his behavior and manner of thinking. He recounts an episode when he tried to be "present" for his wife during a phone call while watching a sporting event.

Therapist: It sounds like you concealed your true wishes, trying to multitask instead of thinking of what you wanted.

Mr. A: Yes, I need to take initiative in the future. That's what I should have done.

Therapist: Yes, though you focus on what to do, what you should have done, not the feeling.

Mr. A: Well, I think we probably could agree upon a time to talk. It's what I'll do from now on.

Therapist: Yes, though again you're not really addressing the issue.

Mr. A [now looking confused, perhaps anxious]: Well, I am good at putting things off [chuckles], though it's different at work. There I'm better at organizing, scheduling things at a moment's notice and so on . . .

Therapist: So again, notice the words, how you're not speaking to how any of this feels. I don't get a sense of what it's like to "schedule at a moment's notice" at work versus the prospect of doing something similar with your wife. You focus on the task, not what you feel as you're doing that.

Mr. A [still looking confused but anxious to please]: How do I feel . . . [pause] I don't know. It's my style to manage this. I wanted to watch it [the sporting event], do what I wanted, and I guess apologize later instead of saying, "can I call you in a while?" . . . so, I don't know [pause]

Therapist: See, if you notice your statement, you might notice inattention to your experience, so you indicate that you don't know how you feel. After several inquiries, you're still finding it difficult to access the discomfort that prevents you asking for what you want.

Mr. A [shaking his head]: It suggests more attention to the game than it does to her.

Therapist: What do you feel as you say that?

Mr. A [without hesitation]: Well, I feel bad. It's not right. Not fair to her. It would be better for me to talk with her about it, work it out, make her number one.

Therapist: Well, here we have some attention to how you feel—guilt, it sounds like—because you didn't do what you believe you should have done. But that's about what followed the action. What's missing still is the feeling that informed *not* talking to your wife, and *not* making her number one, as you put it.

Mr. A [with a further look of confusion]: I guess I'm not getting this. I don't know what feeling you're . . . what feeling other than guilt, if that's what you mean.

Therapist [separating his hands and glancing upward to gesture a mystery without saying what was "meant" which would be too leading]: I'm not sure what feeling . . . as you're not either, which is important.

This vignette depicts a communicative habit presented by many people, but particularly those who act out with addictive behaviors. The passage depicts a confrontation of defense which protects a triadic false self-structure (Masterson, 1976, 1981) that deflects, evacuates, anesthetizes, or intoxicates. However, the interventions abstain from interpreting feeling states, instead observing the habit of not recognizing feelings (even when absence of their expression was pointed out repeatedly). Because Mr. A is not integrating feelings into his relational style, he does not seem like a promising candidate for in-depth therapy. That might not change, at least not in the short term. This indicates a need for a patient approach that speculates about affect upon an understanding of extant ego functioning. A belief that alexithymia (not being in-touch with one's feelings) leads to relapse is axiomatic in recovery circles. Mr. A's inability to express emotions symbolically (via words) is unconscious and may induce relapse in his behavior—seeking prostitutes. Beyond that potential catastrophe, the problem is estrangement from self, plus a dead end with respect to his married life, which Mr. A desperately hopes to improve. But his experience of something not represented in words seems more powerful than his conscious motivation. As a result, after this exchange, attempts to penetrate his defenses were tempered to indicate more broadly that something was missing. His sexual acting out diminished, he reported. He was clear about halting that. Taking this on faith, I sat more quietly with Mr. A, thinking that his fear of impingement—his dread of emptiness—might unfold amid silence, with me. At points of dissociation, a practitioner trained to facilitate affect release with somatic interventions might have directed Mr. A to observe his body for sensations. But psychoanalytic psychotherapy does not displace words in this fashion. Instead, in our framework, we allow something called transference to happen.

A Comment on Psychoanalytic Approaches to Treating Sex Addiction

Notice that the focus with Mr. A was on present stressors, day-to-day experiences that elicited his thoughts and affect, while his OR (familial past) and addiction were held in mind but not explicitly referenced. Contemporary psychoanalysts have largely written about addiction and alcoholism as a phenomenon of discharge-seeking behavior (Director, 2002; Khantzian, 1981; Kohut, 1977a; Waska, 2006) coupled with psychological defenses, reflecting unresolved relational dynamics, frozen object attachments, and poor affect regulation and impulse control. Some nonanalytic observers consider a long-term treatment strategy with sex addicts to be problematic. Within the context of sex addiction, some researchers (Carnes, 2001; Myers, 1995; Seligman & Hardenburg, 2000) have supported the use of a cognitive-behavioral orientation blended with an insight-oriented emphasis; this approach seeks an understanding of the cognitive processes (psychological defenses) that underlie addictive disorders, as well as the influence of past family history. This matches some elements of a psychodynamic approach, as outlined by Shedler (2010) and presented more fully in Chapter 3, but those prescriptions place less emphasis on eliciting affect. And lastly, of course, the course of treatment is designed to be shorter, forestalling a deepening of affect or an intensification of the patient-therapist relationship.

According to Katehakis (2009), because sex addicts have lacked adequate mother-infant relating in upbringings, they are impaired in their right- and left-brain functions of reflection and expression and can therefore tolerate the closeness of therapy only for short periods. She advises an approach that emphasizes mirroring of patient nonverbal states, gaze, and other bodily responses, as well as directing the patient's attention to these sensations as a way to train recognition of disavowed feeling states. In the wearying debate between Balkanized models about treatment efficacy, many consumers still hear that Cognitive Behavioral Therapy (CBT) is the most effective or proven modality with respect to treating addictions. But what elements (specific intervention techniques or formats) of CBT are really proven effective in the treatment of addictive or problem behaviors? What homework assignments best interrupt the distorted cognitions of acting out persons? Do so-called therapeutic separations or honesty agreements work, and how is that determined? Do polygraph exams or full-disclosure exercises lead to positive outcomes for warring couples (however they may be defined or reported)? Also, has it been demonstrated that collateral meetings with fellow professionals facilitate lasting outcomes?

Ironically, addiction specialists who agree that transference dynamics impact treatment outcomes might focus on interventions like therapist self-disclosure (involving the revelation of biographical details about addiction) as a means toward therapeutic alliance. The idea is that therapist self-disclosure either makes their clients more comfortable to reveal their own secrets, or that such disclosures tacitly indicate qualification to treat addiction. This is an opinion, of course. Here's another opinion: troubled individuals project onto helpers a distorted, false-self experience born of historical experience (Masterson, 1981). In therapy, these individuals internalize distortions comprised of ideal, safe, or bad others and bad, unsafe, or ideal selves, and contrary to what some CBT or addiction specialists may assume, they will internalize these projections whether their therapists are behaving as traditional "blank slates" or not. In other words, self-disclosure, being "real" or "human" does not eliminate projections or other defensive postures. As for homework assignments, we think that practice conjures images of high school and the notion that treatment is academic in nature. In addition, when terms like boundaries are invoked, it brings to mind the norms and expectations of play therapy or child analysis: that messes and hurts have to be cleaned up before sessions end. As Furman (1992) wrote, "being understood means being felt and helped to master" (p. 82). Some will accept that being an addict is like being a child and will accept being treated as one for a while, perhaps for the duration of an intensive or residential program. But most won't accept the "I can't but you can" position perpetually, nor should they.

Before Katehakis, Myers (1995) warned against psychodynamic approaches for sex addiction treatment, suggesting that long-term therapy fosters dependence, which becomes contaminated by patterns of domination and submission. In our view, such critiques create more circular arguments: If a person presenting for care meets assessment[6] thresholds for addiction, consumers will likely hear recommendations for intensive and directive interventions to establish

6. In the categories of substance use disorders, the DSM-5 indicates two periods of remission, partial (3 months) and sustained (12 months), in which full criteria for the disorder were previously met, but do not currently remain. These are guidelines that might help determine whether an individual presenting with problem sexual behaviors is sufficiently stabilized such that in-depth psychotherapy can proceed.

structure and foster behavioral stability while not unduly activating stress. Short-term providers may offer educational, cognitive lessons about a patient's developmental history, outlining attachment events and patterns and identifying personality or complex trauma obstacles. Consumers of short-term treatment options might hear that deepened understanding and fuller exploration of underlying issues might occur at a later stage of treatment, but only after stabilization of behaviors. And there may be a follow-up caveat: If an addict is vulnerable to intense affects and prone to acting out as a soothing strategy, then psychodynamic strategies are perpetually contraindicated. Critics of the psychodynamic approach may also claim that personality patterns are immutable and therefore cannot be worked through—a prejudice that Masterson and Kohut sought to dispel—or that addiction is a monolithic state of incapacity, not sufficiently variable to warrant individual approaches.

Coltart (1987) suggested the use of diagnostic interviewing to determine a person's suitability for analytic psychotherapy. Collectively termed "psychological mindedness," the criteria to be evaluated are as follows:

- What is the individual's capacity for self-reflection at a distance from emotional experience?
- Can memories be brought forward with different qualities and affects?
- What is their capacity to tolerate internal reality? Can they distinguish it from external reality?
- Can uncomfortable states of mind be discussed across historical contexts?
- Is there capacity to use imagination, to recognize an unconscious mental life?

Coltart (1987) writes less of transference dynamics, largely because she is describing an interview process. She emphasizes protorelational phenomena, such as the establishment of rapport. In addition, she suggests that a subject's use of metaphor, or sharing of fantasy, can be a useful indicator of capacity. If the person can make tenuous links between psychic (emotional) pain and self-knowledge, then a prescription for an in-depth process may follow. But Coltart concludes that psychoanalytic psychotherapy has nothing to offer those who only wish to be relieved of suffering, echoing Freud and countless others in declaring that transference is the mainspring of analytic work. Transference constitutes an intense, emotional relationship between the patient and clinician that is not accounted for by a presenting problem. Its character ranges from passionate, sensual love to embittered defiance and hatred. Of course, hostility can endanger treatment, but how would a person's whole self be treated if it didn't evoke the fullest range of emotional responses? In the early years of psychoanalysis, transference replaced hypnotic trance as *the* therapeutic phenomenon of care. The idea is that acting out is poured into the treatment, which will absorb the *problem*. So, treatment induces (in both patient and clinician) an experience that recreates the past.

The supposed contraindication of in-depth therapy for those prone to mood or mind-altering behaviors observes states of mind that are not conducive to in-depth thinking. Critics of in-depth approaches seem to think only in terms of initial, crisis, or short-term interventions, or believe that the arrested states of mind of addicts are perpetual or unanalyzable (the term used by psychoanalysts). Basically, short-term providers promote shorter treatment episodes because they are efficient and because they think that addicts can't form relationships. So, in short-term treatment, relationships are only significant referentially. We find this strange because we have found that some of the most "unanalyzable" people in therapy are the most patient or the most tolerant of uncertainty. They discover something in a psychoanalytic framework that speaks to a longing they have not recognized but have at some point felt. And they *can* experience transference. They can have *real* relationships at some point, if they are given a real chance.

In our field, there are many opinions about what addiction is and how it should be treated, with little on these matters proven, which might render all debate about treatment approaches moot. But the following is worth thinking about: if someone assessed as an addict can tolerate closeness or work through relational dynamics over time with a clinician, or *think* in the manner that Coltart or others have outlined, then maybe he's got problems but is not out of control, in danger, or perilous to another. Labels like addiction may stick and inform a path forward, or they may dissolve, and maybe he's not an addict after all.

CHAPTER 2

Sex and Intersectionality

> The cowboy must have spent at least six chaste months on a yoghurt ranch eating nothing but ice cream and buttermilk, and with a water-tight no-handjob clause in his contract. By the time he was through, Juanita looked like the patsy in the custard-pie joke, which I suppose is what she was. The camera proudly lingered as she spat and blinked and coughed . . . Hard to tell, really, who was the biggest loser in this complicated transaction—her, them, me.
>
> —A passage from the Martin Amis novel, *Money*

As the bridge between clinical and public discussions is built, issues of class, sex and gender, and race are superimposed on treatment theories and method. The following is an example of that interconnectedness, commonly referred to as intersectionality: An email in a listserv advertised a workshop and podcast aimed at professionals that purported to teach how to cope with "difficult men." The premise was that an epidemic of malignant narcissism exists among men within our society, with destructive behaviors being passed down from generation to generation, rolling over relationships like a fire in the woods. The language in the advertisement was not unique, although psychotherapists are rarely so yellow, so tabloidal, in public. We doubt that this rhetoric would have been used 50 years ago. A glance at history can reveal how things have changed. When the mental health-care workforce was predominantly male, hysterical women were the target of institutional bias. Psychoanalysis taught that passivity is a feminine trait requiring transformation to an active, assertive (implicitly male) attribute. Fifty plus years ago, life was considered centrifugal; culture might transform expression of a trait such as orality, but that trait was thought to emerge from within as part of human nature. Today, culture, the paradigm of the external, alters that very belief, and as the demographics of our proletariat if not quite our intelligentsia reverse,[1] gender biases reverse, so the narcissistic male replaces the hysterical woman as the poster child of neurotic or personality disorders. Enter sex addiction treatment, the purpose of which is not just to help afflicted individuals with so-called problem behaviors. Its subsidiary aim is to alter masculine ego.

In sex addiction treatment, patients are typically male, and the archetypally betrayed party is an aggrieved wife or girlfriend, seeking to deal with the problem that is *him*. We have treated numerous women who either identify as sex addicts or seem like they might be sex (or love) addicts, but our reflections on their treatment are based less on early, direct assessment of conditions, so they seem less representative. We've had even less clinical experience with members of the lesbian, gay, bisexual, transgender, queer (LGBTQ+) community. Of course, this community is not untouched by sex addiction. The mores that emerge from religious, feminist, divided generational thought, class, or cultural differences about sex are all influential in sex addiction treatment. That said, a heteronormative or cis-gendered male/female binary gets most of the attention in this text.

When we speak to male and female colleagues on matters of sex addiction, discussion often strays from diagnostic criteria to a review of social undercurrents, such as the prevalence of misogyny in contemporary culture. We do not reject the inclusion of such angles, but more often than not, pronouncements seem glib, with unexamined assumptions, and premises expressed as givens. Because the demographics of sex addiction treatment are weighted in favor of men (or not), perspectives seem imbalanced, with assumptions drawn variously from popular culture, religion, science, class, and even mythology.

---

1. According to the American Psychological Association's Center for Work Studies, women comprise 76% of new doctorates in psychology and 74% of early career psychologists. Second, the job research site Zippia.com reports that 70% of therapists in the United States are women.

Sex Addiction: A Cultural Controversy

Let's consider again whether sex addiction is an acceptable term across and beyond professional circles, as something more than a mental health condition. Is it a cultural problem? Is the term appropriately directed at those who regularly use pornography, or frequent houses of prostitution, or otherwise engage in high-risk sexual behavior with multiple, often anonymous partners? As previously indicated, the question is partly medical, but is also ontological (addiction as a state of *being*), moral, and sociopolitical. Some in the field of mental health reject the concept of sex addiction, thinking it an unfairly pathologizing idea; it is a "sex negative" contrivance reflecting a dominant culture religiosity or a patriarchal, traditional family belief system that is more responsible for porn addicts' self-identifications than any frequency of sexual acting out (Grubbs et al., 2014; Hook et al., 2015). Some critics observe that sex addiction theory is an encoded endorsement of monogamy. Implicit in such critiques is a defense of vulnerable social groups, including women and those in the LGBTQ+ community. If the pathology of sex addiction is to be directed at anyone, let it be directed at heterosexual men, some appear to think. Everyone else has already had their share of stigma. However, that stigma may be fortuitous in other respects. "Because gay male culture has been more accepting of sexual promiscuity, it has been easier for gay sex addicts to remain in denial" (Weiss, 2013, p. 90). Due to their traditional ostracism from community, family, and the institution of marriage, gay sex addicts face fewer of the threats that lead straight men into treatment (Weiss, 2013).

Weiss' observation furthers our supposition that close-quarter witnessing of an addictive pattern leverages most interventions, not the addictive patterns in and of themselves. The observation that men represent most of sex addiction treatment admissions is supported by research (Giugliano, 2006; Ley, 2012; Weiss, 2013), with Weiss claiming that 85% of admissions are men. However, such data may be misleading. In a recent survey study involving a nationally representative sample, researchers found that 7% of women and 10% of men reported clinically significant distress or impairment associated with controlling sexual urges or behavior—a far less pronounced disparity in gendered patterns (Dickensen, Gleason, & Coleman, 2018). Also, statistics may track only the stated pretexts for treatment, not the issues that emerge during therapy, and may not reflect the presence of shadow consumers behind those who present for care. For example, a would-be female sex addict might emerge later having entered treatment under the auspices of domestic violence resulting from a discovery of acting out behavior. Still, it's clear that the sex addict label is primarily aimed at men, although this "pathologizing" phenomenon doesn't alter the perception of masculine privilege within the field of sex addiction treatment. Weiss (2013) observed, "The fact is, men who have a lot of sex are usually thought of as studs and players" (p. 83). Is this really a fact? In the context of treatment admission trends relating to sex addiction, such observations appear nonsensical.

Imagine if the demographics of eating disorder treatment were observed with similar inductions. Are women, who represent the majority of admissions to eating disorder clinics, regarded as privileged in that context? Do men find it harder to admit to problems related to eating and weight? Is it therefore society's opinion that women are allowed more freedom than men to eat or to lose or gain weight without judgment from others?

To navigate circular polemics, we must sometimes look beyond logic and consider the unconscious process. According to Freud (1905), an infant's first sexual satisfaction is linked to the intake of food; this suggests that eating disorders disguise sexual neurosis, reflecting loss of an original part-object (the breast). Next, if female sex addiction is more of a taboo than male sex addiction, then the greater numbers of men in treatment would make more sense. The pathologizing of problem sexual behaviors in men constitutes a relative acceptance, or a displacement, meaning identification of one phenomenon as a substitute for another. Male sex addicts, however, shamed they may be when discovered, are acting in general accordance with contemporary (sexist) expectations. Even in a changing social climate, female sex addicts still risk inconceivably shameful exposure, thus consigning them to the proverbial closet. Or, they are strangely heroic, acting in zeitgeist defiance of said expectations.

In collegial circles, much is said about the specter of religion hanging over sex addiction treatment and psychotherapy as a whole. Religion plays or has played an oppressive role in the upbringing of many of our patients, generating guilt as well as isolation. Okay, we've got no dog in this fight, feeling largely neutral about religion, unlike some forefathers of our profession. Age of

Reason giants like Kant (2009) considered religion and revolution (both the contemporaneous French and American varieties) to be obstacles to reasoning. A century later Freud (1913, 1930) followed suit, at least on the matter of religion. However, we wonder if religion serves as a scapegoat for moralists of other kinds today, including practitioners who invoke postmodern ethics, objecting to pornography and prostitution not as sinful entities that compromise marriage or family values, but because they represent exploitation within the context of intimacy and an imbalance with respect to mutual pleasure. Treatment models may echo religiosity by crafting confessional exercises, endorsing the moral stance of impacted spouses, or promoting psychoeducational dogmatism, but they frame sex addiction as a problem of social justice, not religious nonconformity. This pivot from moralism to the ethics of a postmodern Lyceum is perhaps best exemplified by Braun-Harvey and Vigorito (2016), who prefer the term out-of-control sexual behaviors to sex addiction. They also argue for more education about sexuality among mental health practitioners and outline several principles of their Impulsive/Compulsive Sexual Behaviors (ICSB) model, a sexual health framework:

- Consent
- Nonexploitation
- Protection from sexually transmitted diseases and infections and from unintended pregnancies
- Honesty
- Shared values
- Mutual pleasure

These guidelines are meant to distinguish the ICBS model from a framework that conflates sex addiction with paraphilia, or one that subsumes nonconsensual behavior within sex addiction criteria, which risks iatrogenic (treatment-inducing) distress for many in treatment. The ICSB model seeks to reduce biases against specific sexual behaviors, but its cautionary language still casts a wide net of judgment, countering the notion that antisex addiction models are arbitrarily sex positive and are liberally permissive of all sexual activity. The model has an omniscient quality that extols consent between partners; honest communication about motives and the meaning of specific sexual acts; and a spirit of equality that reduces motives of power as it pertains to money, precluding payment for sex. However, it's unclear whether the honesty and shared values guidelines pertain to exclusive relationships and therefore recommend disclosure of behaviors like porn use or attraction to others. Sexual exclusivity is not listed, so presumably "hooking up" is considered ethical in this paradigm, as long as participants give informed consent, make roughly the same amount of money, and only exploit one another's desire.

Sex Addiction and Social Class

The seemingly peripheral issue of class is important for sex addiction, partly because some treatments are expensive, but also because the means of acting out vary depending on individuals' means. As suggested in Chapter 1, some who present for treatment have spent thousands of dollars on prostitutes, generally reflecting affluent lifestyles and freedom of mobility. The same is also true for affair-seeking individuals, who often travel, have legitimate pretexts for spending quantities of cash, or have fluid bank accounts, which enables lying to spouses and others. Due to relative financial freedom, the more affluent sex addict can take time away from work to participate in intensive treatments in the form of residential programs or weekend workshops, spread over days or weeks. Of course, some sex addicts have squandered great sums of money, but their expenditures are usually rivaled or offset by their income-generating capacities. In contrast, the poor man's sex addict is a compulsive masturbator, a user of pornography, or a promiscuous or sexually unconventional figure, but is less likely to be an inveterate consumer of prostitution. Residential retreats or intensive outpatient programs are prohibitively expensive for a working-class person, even if portions of care are covered by insurance because of related mood or behavioral disorders. Even weekly therapy in the form of group or one-on-one sessions may impose a financial burden.

The issue of class also touches on sex offending behavior, at least for lesser dangerous behaviors such as voyeurism or indecent exposure. Consider a young man who has little money, marginal employment prospects, is living with his parents, and has numerous siblings of varying ages plus a grandparent or two, all cohabitating in a cramped living environment. The issue here concerning sex offending or sex addiction is privacy. Where can this young man have sex? Where can he self-gratify? Those who have more space and greater resources take privacy for granted. People present for treatment because they were arrested for masturbating in their cars, or behind fences in public parks. Such men or boys are mandated to sex addiction or sex offender treatment because they have violated the law, not because they have been properly assessed as sex offenders. They are tasked with the challenge of impulse control, and providers like us are meant to help them achieve this reasonable yet discriminatory standard, and while this scenario may not strike you as the most important cultural issue relating to sex, such cases are eye-opening.

Sex Addiction and Gender

On the whole, gender is more divisive than class or ethnicity in today's sex addiction dialogue. While guidebooks and manuals inform the field of sex addiction treatment, a subtext of gender stereotyping pertaining to sexuality shapes psychotherapy, informing or contaminating treatment processes (depending on your point of view). Bemoaning social disadvantage, many theorists and practitioners speak of masculine privilege, referring to men's greater freedom to engage in sexualized behavior without being subject to diminished social status or inordinate shaming. Women incur more physical risk from sexual behavior than men, due to past experiences of sexual abuse that generate ongoing trauma, the threat of sexual assault when entering a dating lifestyle, and the risk of pregnancy if not using protection, a responsibility that also falls into the laps of women. Because women are more likely stigmatized for their sexual activity, commentators assert that women incur more generalized emotional risks, which may be why some practitioners are more reluctant to assign women labels like sex addict. Many assert defining characteristics of women versus men that are echoed in contemporary self-help literature. Consider this example from Alex Katehakis' *Erotic Intelligence*:

> Males and females are attracted to different qualities in one another. When a man sees a beautiful woman, his emotions ride high and his logic disappears. In contrast, females are attracted to a companion who can provide and protect. Thus, when a woman sees an attractive man, she wants to know

> how he thinks and acts, and eventually how he will care for her. Women have larger limbic centers than men. These are emotional networks in the brain that orient women toward caretaking roles like child rearing. Men with high testosterone are more likely to get divorced and have extramarital affairs; men with low testosterone levels are calmer and less aggressive, making them more likely to get married and stay married. (Katehakis, 2010, p. 47)

Since women represent up to 83% of readers of self-help literature (Zhou, 2017), populist thoughts such as these speak to a core readership. Such gender style assignments exist alongside the "men are coming up short" views of authors like Terrence Real (1998, 2003), who argues that men don't avoid intimacy as much as subjugation. He critiques women for being condescending in conflict, suggesting that women err in the manner of their protests, if not in the content of complaints. Real's (1998, 2003) critique of grandiose men who exhibit what he terms "covert shame" seems a fair take on narcissistic defenses, though his implication that men's fear of subjugation is misplaced may not be so fair. After all, if contemporary self-help literature is being written either by or for women, then it is women who are defining the constructs of intimacy and love for present and future society, so men's fear of misrepresentation is legitimate. This recalls what rock music legend Pete Townshend once said of his beloved form: "rock has to say what young people want it to say." As an artist, he understood that he had an audience, but amid the mores-disrupting, social upheaval of rock's halcyon age, also a constituency. The audience demands but also determines truth, and while punditry shapes popular opinion or the trending concerns of artists, the reverse is also true.

There is a great deal of research on gender differences. Based on our experiences, we often find that women seem more sensitive to nonverbal cues in therapy. But in picking apart the views of gender-study luminaries like John Gray, Louanne Brizendine, Steven Pinker, and Simon-Baron Cohen, Cordelia Fine (2010) outlined flawed research practices and debunked much of the science proclaiming innate differences between male and female brains, including differences relating to empathy responses. Also, Eliot et al. (2015) found differences between male and female brains to be minimal, including differences within the hippocampus, which is responsible for memory and emotional responsiveness. The hippocampus had previously been reported as being larger in women than in men, justifying gender stereotypes like "women are more in touch with their feelings." In a meta-analysis of 76 previous studies involving more than 6,000 subjects, this study found that the female hippocampus is *not* significantly larger. Second, the study found that differences in brain size (on average, men's brains are 8% larger than those of women) have no discernible bearing on intelligence or any other specific faculty. Third, the study reported that, contrary to another popular myth, the size of the corpus callosum (a bundle of nerves that connect the two sides of the brain, allowing them to communicate) does not vary according to gender. This is important because we think these myths are still being shared with consumers of psychotherapy, enabling the belief that women possess a superior capacity for empathy or that men are more logical. This in turn inclines clinicians to believe that female sex addicts relate more to the concept of love addiction because sex is not just a biological drive but something that sustains an all-consuming relationship.

As clinicians, we might amplify the stigma argument in one respect: We agree that boys and men are stigmatized if they are *not* actively sexual. However, we challenge other pedantic beliefs. For example, if men are so privileged or "entitled" in their promiscuity, then why are they so secretive about it? Why is the problem the discovery of the behavior rather than the behavior itself? To further this point, we observe that women's envy of privilege is not coupled with admiration of men's promiscuity but with resounding disapproval. This attitude finds its apex in the traction recently afforded the term "toxic masculinity" and in the prevalent use of terms like "creep," "pervert," or "pig" to denote male promiscuity and sexual greed in addition to nonconsensual misconduct, excess assertiveness, and sexual violence.

Something has happened over the last generation (or two or three, perhaps) to reverse a once phallocentric bias. In academic or training institutions, the revolution has come and seems here to stay. *Epater Le Patriarchie*. Meet the new boss. We appear to be living a transitional moment in history in which critiques of female sexual behavior are deemed "slut-shaming" while the lens of insult turns upon men. At the same time, older biases remain, especially if reports about online dating trends are to be believed. Women seem more selective of partners, more observant of safety considerations, and more prone to seeking emotional and physical sparks of intimacy. From these views we extrapolate a corollary: the average man lives just this side of sexual incontinence, and that women are more mature, more holistic in evaluating attractiveness, more "present" in attention to pleasure versus discomfort or pain, and more in tune with nature (in keeping with ancient mythological notions of gender). Meanwhile, to admire white-dressed feminine virtue or reserve is to cosign oppression, so careful men, caught in a sandwich of unacceptable thought, fall silent and withdraw, which appears to nonplus or annoy some feminists. Now, the plights of such men may not matter to an advocate, but unless practicing in a tightly homogenous community, most therapists and other clinicians can't afford to live in a half-object (for example, one-sex) world. They must consider all sides of a story.

It's not clear what psychotherapists should do about prejudice. Training across orientations tends to discourage blunt didacticism, but tacitly encourages views that champion the marginalized and chasten the privileged. Seeking his own "bridge" regarding hateful speech or anti-social beliefs, analyst Donald Moss (2019) wrote, "We are fundamentally uncertain as to whether our consulting rooms should be thought of as public or private spaces. The patient's voice is singular. When that singularity dissolves, when it turns plural, when the language turns against us, overwhelms us, we have no clear recourse. We feel, in effect, 'incited' but can appeal to no court" (p. 327). Clinicians may (consciously or unconsciously) endorse essentialist beliefs, especially stereotypes about men and women. Male patients often refer to women as "more emotional," sometimes with reverent envy, but more commonly with derision. Female patients often ask questions "Why are there so few decent men these days?" or make comments similar to, "Not all of them are like that," in seeming defense of a male society otherwise excoriated in feminine circles. A lonely yet child-seeking woman, having previously heard the advice-lite query, "Have you considered artificial insemination?" might say, "I don't need men, do I?" Saying nothing in response to these expressed biases allows silence to make patients wonder (also, see the mindreading section in Chapter 4). Some of our female colleagues, who report antimale statements by their female clients, seem to take pride in their contentious interventions, thinking themselves egalitarian or pro-social. However, while challenging defeatist thinking, their rebukes leave the premises of their clients' complaints undisturbed. Perhaps they should try silence.

> I once had an unusual opportunity to lead a teenage girls' process group in a group home/hospital setting. The demographics of mental health systems are such that men are rarely placed in positions of care with girls, at least in institutions. But in this instance, with an aberrant dearth of qualified female therapists available, I was asked to lead a twice-per-week process group for as long as six months. The kids in this group home were feral. Splayed across one another, picking at and grooming others' hair and bodies like baboons in the wild, these girls told me which animals they thought their boyfriends resembled. "Dogs," said many of them, laughing. They reserved the terms "creeps" and "perverts" for unattractive yet sexually demonstrative males. "Pigs" was the term preferred by their mothers, though they weren't sure why. Porcine connotes greed, filth, disposability (something to be slaughtered), or possibly power (Orwell's pigs on the farm). These girls didn't seem to regard their boyfriends as greedy or powerful, much less disposable. Instead, they saw them as free, sexually roaming creatures, enviable if somewhat disparaged—disobedient dogs. And they compared stealing one another's dogs to stealing clothes, as if they were morally equivalent acts. I find that most men don't mind the dog epithet; it's the leash that's the problem. The girls didn't seem to think their use of the word dog as hateful or demeaning. Instead, they considered their words a merely playful reflection on male sexuality. Regarding male violence, they seemed ambivalent. They may have been fearful, but some of them were aggressive themselves, and therefore seemed admiring or reliant upon man's militant utility. Helens of Troy, they seemed unaware that a certain brand of prophylactic is marketed at them also.

Today, in mixed company, disgruntled (usually younger) women use terms like "mansplaining" or "sausage party" to protest masculine hubris or the habits of exclusion. The men-as-meat metaphor betrays irony-detection deficits, while "mansplaining" implies that only men are given to insufferable pedantry. Women who use such terms might not know the term misandry, or they might ask, "Is that a thing?" Like their mothers, they'll know the word misogyny, having been raised to observe hate directed at them, not by them.

Mythological Perspectives: The Swine, Virginity, and Scopophilia

Modern mores and neologisms may have turned history on its head. Take our friend the pig, for example. According to Markale (1972), the image of the pig is associated with the female in Celtic and Greek mythology. It underlies the myth of Aphrodite, one of the oldest goddesses of the Hellenic world (the prefix *Aphro* is related to the Latin *Aper*, meaning "wild boar"). Male fantasies transformed the figure of the sow goddess, repressing its divine meaning (prosperity and love) to leave behind sexual images connected with blood and corruption.[2] So, a transformed "swine" is someone who practices abnormal fornications, and the "dirty man" (now the sty inhabitant) fantasizes about implicitly degenerate women.

In the feminine mythos, primitive society was once matriarchal, reflecting women's exalted link to nature and procreative forces: Mother Earth (or Gaia in Greek mythology). The emergence of patriarchal society submerged feminine icons, hence women's common links to water and caves: the Lady of the Lake in British folklore, and the Japanese goddess Ame-no-Uzume, who lured the sun out of a cave. For men, woman represents the ancient ocean, or that to which men crave a return: a moist, original womb (sex as a reversal of birth). The ocean metaphor parallels the original state of the earth before dry land emerged. The feminine sun created light and life; the lunar male arose later. In usurping Mother Earth, man asserted his freedom, but if woman was as free in her sexuality as man, it would endanger patrilineal succession, for how would men know if they were the fathers of children born to sexually free women? A modern rationalist might point out that such concerns are antiquated because we now have contraception and paternity

---

2. Frazer (1981) wrote that, across various cultural legends, the seclusion of girls at puberty reflects a dread of menstruation, plus a primitive belief that women are impregnated by the sun. Therefore, they are charged with a powerful force which, if not kept within limits, may prove destructive to all that they touch.

testing techniques. But the point of myth is to illuminate (some say reduce) thought that traverses time and scientific progress—in this case, man's lingering distrust of the feminine.

Some blame biblical scripture for patriarchal and sexual privilege in Western culture. Contrary to Freudian theory, in scripture the evil of man is not a phylogenetic[3] given, but rather the stuff of creationist myth: the sin by the first man and woman of eating the forbidden fruit from the tree of knowledge, with Eve blameworthy because she gave the fruit to Adam. "Eve was framed" reads a bumper sticker that adorns the cars of many of Eve's outraged descendants. Also, consider Ephesians 5:22: "Wives, submit yourselves to your own husbands as you do the Lord." In other words, scripture placed husbands in charge. Women often quote this text to gird their protests against male privilege. They blame the sanctioning of submission for the thwarting of career aspirations and sexual freedom by the masculine order. Additional text from Ephesians 5:25 is not quoted as often: "Husbands, love your wives, just as Christ loved the church and gave up his life for her." In other words, men may be on top, but they're meant to sacrifice themselves and take physical risks to protect women whereas women take physical risks to protect children. The sacrifice they make for men is psychological: a sacrifice of voice and identity as beings separate from men. Over time, we observe the result of these arrangements: the condoning of everything from prostitution to porn use, to infidelity, to wage inequity, and—most unfortunately—to varying degrees of sexual abuse.

Mythology-like metaphor, dreaming, and arts are a condensing path to the unconscious through which scholars glean the organization of societies, both past and present. Of course, religion has an impact. Biblical tradition organizes symbols into values that deliver notions of sinfulness, virginity, and forbidden pleasures, which empower reactionary entities like the porn industry. Also, so-called

---

3. In biology, phylogenetics pertains to evolutionary development of a species. In Freud's (1913) Darwinian-styled theory, man inherits his sexual/aggressive and incestuous wishes from the primal horde, or early man. Uninterested in modern religion, Freud thought man's original trauma (sin?) was the murder of a tribal elder, plus incest; the subsequent cannibalizing of that *body of the father* was not the sacrament it later became.

wedding night virgin-testing exists across cultures. In some cases, the red stain on the white dress is displayed publicly to demonstrate a bride's purity. In others, the bedsheets are inspected after the wedding night to verify the status of the virgin.

Porn often exploits virginity by casting objects of envy and desire as virgins: boys who are especially excited before their first time, and girls who are especially attractive because their cleansed, even prepubescent virginity, implied by the waxed or bald pubis, is ripe to be despoiled or claimed. A religious objection to porn focuses on the sinfulness of promiscuity, sex outside a consecrated marriage. A feminist objection refers more specifically to the reduction of women to physical objects, or at least to figures under the control of male authority. As this mirrors a societal norm, porn becomes a microcosm of misogyny. Misogyny, in contrast to misandry, is not deemed a reaction to extant social norms, but rather an unconscious yet powerful reaction to an original, prehistorical truth that exists in the minds of all men: that women, or at least one woman (mother), was once in charge of everything.

The virgin mythology relates further to the question of sexual double standards and lends credence to the stigma assigned to female sex addicts in particular. The masculine yearning for virgins is rarely given a sound rationale. Some speculate that it reflects a need to control women or a search for an unrealistic ideal, or a special discomfort aimed at female promiscuity because virginity can't be redeemed. Once lost, the innocence and perfection that virginity represents are gone forever, so the sexualized woman becomes "damaged goods." Freud (1912) coined the term Madonna-whore complex to represent the male dilemma: he cannot love a desired figure, and he cannot desire a loved or respected figure because of Oedipal prohibitions against incest and the consequent fear of castration. Therefore, he splits his affection and desire. Postpuberty, he may seek a nurturing female partner, but this nurturing quality activates repression of the forbidden desire. Alternatively, angry at the lost object, he may take revenge against the "weaning" mother via sadistic attitudes toward replacement women. The designated "whore" or the spectrum of pornographic fantasies serve as receptacles for otherwise denied impulses, which spares him from the dilemma, or so he may unconsciously believe. Considered in addiction terms, virginity—unlike sobriety—cannot be recovered when lost, but it can be revisited and despoiled, repeatedly, with interchangeable objects or fantasies.

Later, lesser-known theories reformulated Freud's theory of castration anxiety into sexual neuroses indicating fear of losing the genitals that are actually possessed. Drawing on the work of Karen Horney (1924, 1926), Elizabeth Mayer (1985) wrote about women's psychological attachments to the vulva and clitoris. A woman's "opening" represents her potential for inner space, a capacity lost by the male sex. Men are "closed over" via their genitalia, yielding an unreceptive mind or lack of emotional depth ("Something's wrong with *him*," she complains). This theory parallels the phallocentric theory more commonly associated with psychoanalysis, not to mention those tropes of male pathology replete within self-help literature. According to Mayer (1985), women who exhibit genital anxiety act with duplicity like that of men who place women on idealized pedestals only to demean or subjugate them. Such women seek out men who are caricatures of masculinity, not because they idolize a masculine ideal, but to be reassured of their own feminine qualities, which they deem superior. However, such qualities may render women vulnerable. Because they fear that male caricatures might excite them sexually, they employ the feminine talent of keeping that excitement within, of not *showing*. Excitement is for men to show, on the outside.

Modern mythopoeic art doesn't need porn scenarios to express misogyny and other prejudices. Far more potently, modern films, including mainstream films,[4] as well as other mediums of popular art, convey the attitudes of men and women toward one another. For baby boomers, there are perennial ladies' men, like the character James Bond, or the actors James Stewart or Cary Grant in . . . well, pick a Hitchcock film, or the sullen ramblings of blues singers or their rock and roll derivatives. The same goes for popular culture today. As pundits routinely draw attention to scopophilic

4. This author's favorite satire of hypermasculinity is the 1964 black comedy film, *Dr. Strangelove or: How I Learned to Stop Worrying and Love the Bomb*. Phallic images of sex and aggression, the death instinct, and the objectification of women abound, and underlie the film's plot: An air force general named Jack Ripper(!) is obsessively fearful that the nation's water supply is contaminated, poisoning "precious bodily fluids"; he blames communism (not masturbation?). Because he was impotent during love-making, he launches a nuclear attack on the Soviet Union.

media, misogynistic lyrics in rap or pop music that cast women as untrustworthy, mean, or disloyal-to-the-core "bitches" or "whores" (think Kanye's "Gold Digger"), the television and film industry's casual misandry tends to fly under the radar of intellectual scrutiny. Think of those innumerable depictions of men as mindlessly sexual beings who pursue women with aggressive, objectifying intent—so oblivious to good manners, romance, or the need for genuine intimacy that women might just as well abandon men and choose one another instead (think Ariana Grande's "Thank You, Next"). The attitudes justifying such characterizations are reactionary: because they represent the *truth* of women's experiences, they are condoned by apologists.

Modern myths coincide with modern values to convey morality and protect institutions. Undercurrents filter down into therapists' offices, lurking as assumptions that inflect counsel. Like any culturally relevant phenomena, assumptions about an addict's capacities for greed, envy, or hate are of clinical interest. Therefore, misogyny is relevant to sex addiction because observers are insistent about it. The men in our practices sometimes address the topic of misogyny, often missing the point of complaints by shrugging and saying things like, "I love women, so sue me." In making statements like this, they mean to express their enjoyment of women's physical beauty, or of flirting with women who are considered fun or agreeable. This is about wanting women, not loving them, which may be a matter of what is conscious and what is not. Bader (2009) observed in his male patients an ironic motivation when using porn, even in its most demeaning forms: a loving, if not respectful wish to protect women from impinging, unacceptable desires, and one's self from guilt. The secret-keeping, denial, and even violent fantasies experienced vicariously through porn are meant to discharge yet contain aggressive sexual feelings, to avoid triggering their release through horrific acts like rape.

By pointing out that those who become addicted to porn or prostitution do not become violent criminals in vast numbers, Bader (2009) contests the common belief that addictions, or sex addiction in particular, are progressive or life-threatening. Echoed by Ley (2012), Bader's observation is supported by a research review that found a link between higher porn use and lower rates of rape and sexual assault (Ferguson & Hartley, 2009). By implication, porn is an outlet, a "maintenance program," as some patients put it, or a tool that (literally) climaxes and therefore terminates desire, which protects self and others from dreaded harm. Conversely, health professionals describe allostasis as a process by which the body responds to stressors to regain homeostasis.

Alternatively, consider the following take on objectifying voyeurism: Ogden (2005) described a male patient who reflected on a childhood memory of molesting his sister ("playing doctor" as it is euphemistically termed): "His repeatedly looking into his sister's genitals seemed to me to represent an attempt to find out what was 'in there' (inside his mother's body and mind), which was at once 'grotesque' and with amazing powers" (p. 18). In Ogden's analysis, the patient's gaze into his sister's "privates" is less a precocious pleasure than a wondrous inspection of the elusive feminine, a fantasy/horror dating back to preverbal experience. In addition, this is an expression of inadequacy; the patient felt that he was invisible to his mother and that women as a whole were unknowable.

Analysts have been making these kinds of observations and in effect writing about pornography for over a century, beginning (again) with Freud (1909). What he termed scopophilia in reference to his famous "Rat Man" case, variously called the scopophilic instinct or scopic drive, refers to a "burning desire to look"; in particular, it refers to the seeking and discovery of a penis or lack of one. Lacan (1938, 1953) referred to this instinct or drive (the latter adding psychology to the biological construct of the former), assigning desire to a "Mirror Stage" of infant development. In this stage, the child aims for the look of desire in gazing at the mother, who may look at him as he sees himself; at some point she becomes a lost object. Fetishes may also represent lost objects, substituting items that conceal genitals (underwear), or a *last part-object seen* (legs, feet) before eyes and scopic drive once settled upon the forbidden. So, what we commonly think of as mindless voyeurism is an imaginary way to understand the desire of the other. From the perspective of a heterosexual man, it expresses the desire for women who replace the mother from whom he was weaned. She can be replaced, but never completely, and the obsession that defends against this loss never fully satisfies. This dreamy theory of male/female separation further recalls the myth of Psyche and the god Eros: Eros longs for his forbidden woman, but can only visit Psyche at night in a secret hideaway that he provides; although she is lonely and longs for him as well, he must remain invisible to her.

CASE ILLUSTRATION: VOYEURISM (MR. B)

The following is an exchange with a man whose initial disclosures were vague but admitted to regularly objectifying women in both public and private settings. It reflects a difference in approach from the case of Mr. A described in Chapter 1. Here, a discovery of sexual acting out is not the stated pretext of treatment:

Mr. B: That woman I mentioned—I couldn't reach her. Sometimes I voyeur when that happens. I take pictures, in secret. I feel weak, you know?

Therapist: What do you mean?

Mr. B: I never have a chance with her. I feel so drawn to it. They [the women?] impress me.

It's tempting during this session to begin a Q&A, a belated assessment protocol, but shifting to a Q&A would reflect a medical—not a psychodynamic or analytic—sensibility: taking care of the patient by collecting data about symptoms, and proceeding with a treatment plan based on a diagnosis. What's the problem with this approach? Shifting abruptly to a position of assessment would constitute a defensive enactment (a variation on repetition compulsion), as it may pull the therapist into the role of voyeur, given the projective potential at this moment: "Really, tell me what you saw. What did you do with the pictures?" Does this mean that an assessment opportunity should be forsaken? No. Some details of this man's acting out were revealed, though not because I asked after them abruptly or directly. Instead, keeping an analytic frame, I tried an interpretation that spoke to the live experience:

Therapist: Let's notice that you've told me one or two things that you're calling voyeuring, but that's all you've said about it. It sounds like an invitation for me to know this about you . . . and at the same time, maybe it's something you don't want me to know.

Observe the themes of perfection-seeking and loss-avoidance in Mr. B's "dream girl" reverie in our next session:

Mr. B: If I look, it lowers my self-esteem. I feel it. I feel like dirt. I had this idea that my sponsor supported. [By this time, he's informed me that he regularly attends SAA.] Talk to her, he said. Talk to the girl. Be upfront . . . she's a real person. So, I did. I talked to her and realized that she is a real person, you know?

Therapist: You mentioned self-esteem. How was that affected by talking to her?"

Mr. B: It made me feel courageous. It made me feel good. But . . . if I see her—see her again—I'd feel compelled. I want to talk to her again.

Therapist: You seem disturbed.

Mr. B: [Running a hand through his hair] I'm afraid of missing out.

Therapist: Missing out on what?

Mr. B: I don't know . . . on being friends, or [chuckles] more voyeuristic opportunity, I guess. She's my dream girl. Not the first time I've been there, I know [alluding to previous "dream girls"]. She's my . . . she's my fantasy. [Pause] I feel compelled. It's so powerful.

Therapist: Powerful?

Mr. B: It can destroy. So, you know, I think about her, masturbate. Move on. It relieves.

Therapist: When you say destroy, what's that like?

Mr. B: Fear. If I do this, if I keep doing this, I'm not gonna accomplish anything. I'm gonna lose . . . it makes me feel strange.

Therapist: Sounds like . . . when you act upon these feelings . . . when you act upon "feeling compelled". . . you don't like who you become.

Mr. B: You think I'm strange, too? [A projective moment]

Therapist: I'm saying you end up not liking how *you* feel . . . about yourself.

This response touches on a psychoeducational comment that I'm sometimes inclined to make: While addictions make people feel good, they don't make people feel good about themselves. That difference is crucial.

Mr. B: [Shifting uneasily on the couch] Yeah, though . . . I don't know. I sometimes think I should go for it, you know? I think of the woman I told you about, that I met when I was younger. The broken heart. I mean, I broke her heart, I know, because she turned out to be a bitch. But at first, she was like a dream girl, and I was proud of that dream, of being with her. And this girl . . . she's like that, only I think better. She's real. [Shrugs]

[Pause]

Therapist: I think that something was stirred a few moments ago. I think that when I said you don't like how you feel about yourself, you experienced discomfort. [Pause] Seems you felt something missing. You had one of those "missing out" moments.

Mr. B: You know, it's weird you say that. I didn't think that—what you said—but I had some kind of feeling, like an empty feeling. It was uncomfortable, like you said.

This passage reveals something important about Mr. B's thoughts and feelings about women. Despite his anger, he passively retreats from them. The passage also reveals the potential for an analytic process. Despite having less time away from his acting out behaviors (he may not yet be "sober," as that term is used in 12-step circles) than Mr. A, Mr. B displays a greater capacity to think about his problem, observe his experience, and lament objectifying women. Because he seems more flexible, alive, and interactive in his treatment, and less dissociative, he can make better use of the psychodynamic approach illustrated here. The differences between Mr. A and Mr. B bring to mind what is sometimes discernible about a person's early development: An individual who was once more or less integrated in his capacities but regressed in what he brings to treatment is different from someone who seems unintegrated as a baseline condition. Winnicott (1952, 1960) described the latter as "never held" in a state of omnipotent illusion, and thus completely unintegrated in his thoughts and actions.

Hate, Objectification, Exploitation, and Male Sacrifice

The psychological blend of sex and aggression is an important side topic or subtext of sex addiction treatment. To discuss it properly, gender bias about aggression and hate must first be addressed. In contemporary culture, the hate that women express toward men (misandry), whether they are sex addicts themselves or partners of sex addicts (or not identifying as either), is considered outrage rather than hate. This difference is crucial because hate is generally considered endogenous, unjust, and primal.

Misogyny seems linked to a developmental task during which a boy must separate from the mother to whom he was once physically attached. According to Stoller (1968), this merger with the maternal figure is life's incipient fusion, which forges identity (a "proto-feminine" gender identity), and his contention that gender identifications result from a separation-individuation stage of development further implicates so-called hyper-masculine behaviors. As the saying goes, it's not the same for girls. Fathers are not physically attached at a nascent age, so a girl's separation from the opposite-sex figure is less intense, rupturing, and primal, and also less suggestive of an original taboo.[5] A girl's unconscious desire is to reach out for that detached male figure, not to pull away disparagingly, as boys typically do from their engulfing mothers.

Of course, boys don't have a monopoly on oppositional anger. Girls and women often separate from mothers and fathers with what seems like similar vehemence, but few would lecture them about misandry or toxic femaleness when they do so. The story of women's protest is framed as an appeal to an inattentive, unavailable male figure or institution. Women cry foul at aggression, sexual bullying, and social disregard, but don't consider their outrage hateful. They think it just, or even loving. So, women don't hate men, because the concept of trauma renders hate exogenous. Correspondingly, the word misandry isn't widely known because its use appears to critique feminine anger, which the repression barriers of today's society do not countenance. Therefore, "man-hating," a slang term that does critique feminine anger, substitutes for misandry in pop culture, though it languishes as nonestablishment thought, dodging academic oversight. From an analytic framework, misandry derives from a splitting defense: it is hatred *of* men, but also the vigilant assignment of hate *to* men. This relegates masculine dissent to the void of dismissible thought, which is why those who plaintively use the word misandry are cast as antifeminist by progressive orthodoxy. Outrage, as platformed anger, lives in conscious,

---

5. The pedigree of this view lies in Freud (1905), but more prominently Klein (1928). Klein's theory asserted that a male infant abandons oral and anal positions, altering the aim of his libidinal position to one of penetration, though he retains his love-object, the mother. The female infant carries over from oral to genital stages a receptive aim, retaining a libidinal position, but she changes her love-object to the father. It is left to opinion to determine which sex faces the more complicated task, or how this formulation might fit a nonheteronormative premise.

living memory, is publishable and inspires the white noise of a righteous crowd, but it doesn't govern how everyone thinks. So, without asserting moral equivalence or symmetry—terms invoked to block expression not meeting these thresholds—toxic femininity, if deemed a thing, might be framed as a passive tendency, because rebuking women's aggression might "turn back the clock." Well, clocks go round and round, we might notice.

At the same time, men's sexual behavior (and aggression) is often taken at face value because it appears to reflect greater freedom and is often perceived in facile terms as a function of innate biological drive. Sexual acting out is pleasure-seeking behavior, not an investigative gaze into the feminine mystique, or a protest against an unjust system, or a dissociative act ("He's not an addict, he's just a dick!"). Others regard men's sexual freedom through a social lens. Man's seeming prerogative to seek gratification outside of marriage is a privilege that is linked to greater social responsibility. This reflects a traditionalist perspective, tacitly delivered in polite society, or more explicitly so in male-only circles. From a slightly more progressive view, sexual entitlement is seen as a function of social advantage, a reward for assuming society's sacrificial and therefore acceptably aggressive role. Farrell (1999) refers to this as the "women and children first" principle, which renders men disposable, like their namesake pigs. On the related topic of narcissistic needs, Giugliano (2006) observes that sexually addicted men yearn for admiration and mirroring, act out to relieve inadequacy, and—in greater numbers than are known—reenact episodes of childhood sexual abuse. Giugliano goes on to suggest that if narcissistic wounding is such a prominent feature of sex addiction, a psychodynamic self-psychological approach such as that advanced by Kohut (1971, 1977b), rather than a denial-confronting addiction model, is indicated for treatment.

Voyeurs act out feelings, like aggression, that they split off (or dissociate). To support this thesis, we must depart from dry theories of pornography that highlight the transiency of performer interactions and their detached, self-gratifying, uncaring attitudes, but demur on the nitty-gritty truth. The acting in porn has never been great—no kidding—but this doesn't mean that porn doesn't have meanings that betray the varied wishes of consumers. Consider time-tested porn scenarios involving women being lured into sexual situations with authority figures, usually with an undercurrent of blackmail. A supposed landlord approaches an apartment door, rings the bell, and waits for a female resident to open up. The girl who appears will become the performer of the following scene, but first there will be dialogue and a semblance of a plot: The girl's rent is late, but she is down on her luck and cannot provide the necessary funds; what's a girl to do? That question hangs suggestively while the chuckling landlord is invited inside, ostensibly to discuss the matter further. Because the rest, which proceeds as you might imagine it, constitutes the dominant portion of the scene, you might wonder why the skit-like opening is even necessary. On the surface, it isn't necessary, but it instills in the viewer's mind a fantasy beyond the physical aspects of sex in which an average guy, who implicitly cannot get laid under ordinary circumstances using charm or looks, gets lucky with an eager, sexually greedy woman whose economic disadvantage he can exploit. Sometimes, even for the presumably unthinking porn user, a filmmaker must provide interesting reasons for why people are having sex.

Imagine the previous commentary as a voiceover for a porn scene, or as one of those DVD "extras" features that accompany popular films. Viewers might hit the mute button, thinking it a buzz-kill, or complain, "you're overthinking this," because some things are not meant to be thought about. We disagree, of course, and think killing the buzz with thought ought to be part of treatment. When we discuss scenarios like the one just described, our patients recognize the features and acknowledge porn's power and exploitation subtext. However, they also perceive power dynamics that crisscross the gender divide, rejecting the belief that male subjugation is oxymoronic. Here's another common porn scenario: a coolly arrogant seductress services one or more subservient partners, manually or orally stimulating them but not receiving any physical stimulation herself. It can be inferred that her satisfaction stems from the ease with which she can inspire climax from a gathering of faceless men, which reflects her sexual prowess, not theirs. During the sex that follows, the players do not writhe in passionate, sensual heat; instead, their movements are jerky, sweatless, and predictably choreographed. Would those who decry the singular objectification of women in porn revise their theses after watching a scene like this? Might they concede that the implicit qualities of porn demean everyone involved, rendering the standard narratives about porn hackneyed, one-sided, or just uninteresting?

Probably not. For some, the "seductress" scene might still be cast as male neurosis or fantasy that objectifies women regardless of which performers affect superior airs or positions. This is because superiority is not judged, shall we say, equally. For example, a man kneeling before a woman is an act of romantic supplication, or possibly a sexual submission—either is a transient departure from a privileged role. A woman kneeling before a standing man is less romantic, connoting crude subjugation of an already vulnerable person, assuming group identity standards. Same behavior, different meaning. So, in porn, men are positioned in upright, soldierly poses while a camera zooms in on a smiling female gaze, and those smiles persist beyond climax, holding on until the last drop of an ejaculatory "facial" has been squeezed out. Is she grossed out like the average porn hater? Is she unhappy? No, implies the filmmaker. She is smiling, signifying her approval of her partner's performance and acceptance of the (implicitly male) voyeur watching this performance. What does the female actor internalize from the man's postcoital satisfaction? Revisiting Giugliano (2006) may cause us to wonder what the male actor internalizes, or whether the voyeur really feels his self-esteem "restored," even temporarily, by watching this degrading act. If this is a power dynamic, then who has won?

The meaning of objectification bears scrutiny not because it's wrongly applied to pornography and prostitution, but because the term's popular meaning has become stereotyped, like the concept of addiction. According to a feminist perspective, originally influenced by Kant's writings on dignity and humanity, persons who are objectified are demeaned, rendered invisible, or else reduced in purpose. Dworkin (1991) broadly observed that when persons are turned into a thing or commodity or are bought and sold, they are rendered less human. Langton (1993) wrote of pornography's "assumed objectivity," referring to men's false belief that women *want* to be submissive, while MacKinnon (1987) posited that, via porn, women exist only to the end of male pleasure (sex is over when he climaxes). More recently, Levy (2005) paraphrased OR theory, suggesting that women internalize the male gaze and participate in "raunch culture" by self-objectifying. Therefore, in feminist society, heterosexual man is Uranus, ever raping or cannibalizing women. Or he is Orpheus, perhaps clever and adoring, but ever consigning poor Eurydice to the underworld with his thoughtless gazing. We agree, sort of, but also consider these views tired and scotomized. Recall, for example, that in OR theory the term "object" denotes *other*; the term part-object refers to a thing (and most specifically, breast or penis); that Klein (1935) theorized of all infants that a relation to part-objects springs from a phantastic and unrealistic nature of a child's relation to objects and to parts of a child's own body and surrounding people and things, which are dimly perceived. Recall our supposition that porn addicts do not experience sex in the self. To objectify is to reduce to a thing or a fantasy, to place attributes in others, and to hate one's sexuality as much as anyone else's. Sexual stimuli are coveted yet deemed onerous or unattainable, and better to experience from afar.

Empirical research into objectification may further confound an average view of the concept, or its applications. In a study by Bernard, Gervais, and Allen (2012), researchers presented participants with pictures of near-naked men and women in sexualized poses on computer screens. The pictures were presented right side up and later upside down, with participants asked to match them. The participants were better able to match the pictures of men than those of women, suggesting that the women in the pictures were more likely viewed as physical objects, and that men are recognized by their faces and not by their underwear or other body parts. The men are individualized, presumably because faces are more individually distinctive than, say, buttocks. This study was published within a commercial article, bridging research and wider social discussion with the hyperbole, "Objectification of women is a real, measurable problem" (Bernard et al., 2012). If this specific distinction—being recognized by one's face—does *not* constitute objectifying behavior, then the concept seems loosely defined. If you accept that gazing at faces is less demeaning than ogling other body parts, then we have heuristic (or at least culture-bound) criteria for healthy gazing. But how does this distinction measure whether an individual is being assessed by psychological criteria rather than aesthetics? In other words, how does the study support what Katehakis (2010) suggests: that women see an attractive man and venture thoughts as to the nature of his mind, whether he will be an adequate partner and so on? It seems that such research, which implies scientific underpinnings to its conclusions, contains interpretive leaps aimed at an overly credulous consumer base.

Studying the gendered content of online pornography, Klaassen and Peter (2015) analyzed the top 100 most viewed videos from four of the world's most popular porn sites: Pornhub, Redtube, YouPorn, and XHamster. Coding over 100 hours of professionally produced heterosexual porn, these researchers noted indicators of objectification, power, and violence. They found that there were more close-ups of female body parts and more images that focused on male pleasure. However, they also found that women and men were equally likely to be initiators of sexual activity and that close-ups of female faces outnumbered those of male faces, suggesting the privileging of masculine gaze, though the meaning of this seems ambiguous.[6] With respect to power, videos were no more likely to depict males in positions of higher social status than females. In terms of sexual dominance and submission, approximately half of the videos exhibited no gender differences, while the other half depicted males in dominant positions. Few videos depicted nonconsensual sex, but those that did were equally likely to depict males and females as victims. This study doesn't represent all internet porn, but the findings suggest that the industry is not what it used to be. Although sex or gender inequality still exists, exploitation of both men and women is apparent in contemporary pornography.

Regardless, the concept of exploitation as it relates to pornography and prostitution is skewed because Western society seems sensitive to exploitation only when it pertains to sex. On the whole, our society is more devoutly consumerist than religious. So, do we pause when the products we consume are manufactured on the backs of the poor and enslaved or perpetrate harm because of toxins like Mica (used for electronic products and makeup)? Politicians do little to contest a system of usury, unregulated business, and pay inequity that yields wide gulfs between rich and poor, but they'll vote quickly to outlaw sexual misbehavior. In 2014, for example, the California legislature voted unanimously (72-0) to pass bill AB1775, which adds the viewing of sexual material depicting minors over the internet to categories of behavior that must

6. Our thoughts on this are mixed: we think the researchers' inference is that this disparity constitutes objectification of men as they are rendered impersonal. However, the conscious point of this maneuver, especially in amateur porn, is likely to protect the privacy of the male performer.

be reported as child abuse. Written by the California Association of Marriage and Family Therapists (CAMFT), which sheepishly informed its membership about the bill a month before its passage, AB1775 is grounded in a pair of dubious pretexts: (1) reporting of internet users by informant therapists will mitigate child abuse, and (2) individuals seeking treatment for the compulsive use of pornography, including that depicting minors, do not warrant confidentiality rights. AB1775 was recently presented before the California Supreme Court—the result of a lawsuit brought forth in part by our colleague, Don Mathews—only to be sent back to lower courts so that its assumptions could be studied further.

Let's put this in context. As a society, we pay for violence in its military and policing forms. We also patronize violence by viewing fascistic action films or gladiator sports. Our domestic media pays far more attention to human trafficking with respect to prostitution than the recruitment of boys into paramilitary gangs in war zones within emerging economies. And amid the COVID-19 crisis, we pay for some to risk their lives just to buy us groceries. The consumer is complicit in economic oppression and violence, but when it comes to sex, we are doubly parochial, prurient, and, in layers, hypocritical. In American society, we disdain payment for sex more than anything else. We'll pay for just about any human need if an exponent's expression is restrained, but we don't protest exploitation of athletes or laborers nearly as fiercely as we do that of sex workers. Why? The religious among us say that sex is sacred and should be treated as such by legal systems and the arts. But is this why the vastly nonreligious, the polyamorous, or sexual health experts think prostitution is wrong? Sexual health experts argue that sex work is a public health risk. But many legal jobs are dangerous and incur (proportionally) more workplace deaths or injuries as far as we know. No, exploitation in and of itself isn't the reason that porn and prostitution stir social justice ire. Progressive society half-thinks that sex is too personal to commercialize, but many in its midst are merely elitist: they believe that sex calls for effort and talent, so porn and prostitution users are lazy, sexually inadequate, or guilty of sexual cowardice. We think psychoanalytic theory reflects a more basic, if half-conscious complaint: sports and work sublimate sex and death whereas porn and prostitution consummate, and consummation blended with work breaks superego rules. It misses the point of sublimation.

Because women (generally) do not pay for sex, or because their male partners are presumptively consensual, women's misandrist motives are given a clement glance by the progressive society that inhabits psychotherapy's vanguard. As suggested in Chapter 1, we believe this pass extends to FSLA treatment, even though the jargon of sex addiction treatment doesn't quite fit social justice principles. Consider a concept like perpetration: in treatment circles, this term does not necessarily refer to violent sexual offending or prostitute-seeking, but rather to any sexual acting out behavior coupled with gaslighting. Perpetration is an abusive betrayal of a trusting other, comprised of gaslighting behavior plus the inducement of reality-ego fragmentation (Minwalla, 2012). Perhaps some female sex addicts are being told that their acting out is a perpetration of trauma on others, though we doubt it somehow. That would violate the currently popular, "*Girl*, stop apologizing," dictum or its decades' old predecessor, "You go, girl!" Although women's sexual acting out may betray, demean, or gaslight others, including men, it is generally cast as self-objectification. This legitimate, if selective, application of OR theory spins perpetration rhetoric, offering support to some acting out men but probably more so to women. (Internalized misandry? No, not a thing.) This results in confrontations from providers like, "You're selling yourself short [with acting out behaviors]," or "The person you're really harming is yourself."

Would such observations kill the buzz of a habitual porn user or someone who engages in some other problem behavior? Would it make for a real, if not-exactly-polite discussion of all that is objectifying or raunchy?

> A man speaks about his affinity for bondage themes, so-called BDSM (bondage/discipline, dominance/submission, sadism/masochism). As he catches my eye, I notice him twitch. He pauses and volunteers, "It's not about power," exhibiting the preconscious defense of negation, as if guessing at my thinking about him. "It's something else," he suggests—something he doesn't name [his own subjugation, reversed versus accepted?].
>
> A female patient reveals a similar penchant for BDSM. "I kinda liked it," she says shyly, understating her interest yet experimenting with revelations. Next, she muses ruefully that she has let herself be used and worries more explicitly about my judgment of her.

These examples exhibit compelling transference moments that relate to gender narratives: despite his negation, the man conceptualizes his BDSM partner only as a victim (or not). The woman's BDSM partner is conceptualized as a perpetrator despite her consent, or he is irrelevant; her experience, within her acting out episode or her enactment with me, is either self-contained or bound with an abstracted other. It, meaning he (or she), hides a lot and has ways to feel better if not good about one's self. This impaired self might as well be termed an "it" and further subordinated to others' needs. So, family and other loved ones must be attended to materially, or otherwise protected from the ugly truth that the "it" presents. This is Frankenstein thinking: off to the Arctic he goes, exiled yet sacrificing, protecting others' feelings and his fragile ego simultaneously. Paradoxically, the acting out figure betrays an unworthy self-image by acting out a guilty pleasure that should always be kept out of sight, just as the self should be kept out of sight.

The male sacrifice/doghouse exile, based on the war ethos that he who is sacrificing is privileged to act out, is of course antiquated. In the 21st century, it is no longer necessary for the average man to prepare for war, especially in the Western world where a post-nuclear reality has rendered mass conventional warfare obsolete. Depending on class or race, the call for muscle by the infrastructure or security needs of our modern society, or the effects of oxytocin, which in males may facilitate aggression toward or avoidance of the antisocial (Gao, Becker, & Kendrick, 2016), man may remain at risk. But not the levels of risk that his forebears endured, so modern man must adapt. Markale (1972) opined the following: "masculine society is aggressive and must submit to a peaceful transformation by women and what they stand for. Then it will finally be able to free itself of the taboos besetting it" (p. 255). Make love, not war. The taboos mentioned by Markale allude to Oedipal mythology (Freud, 1924): man's obsession with forbidden sex (incest) and not-so-forbidden war. Second-wave feminists like Markale, the seminal Friedan (1963), or the later Benjamin (1990), seemed to look over their shoulders at Freud, who observed aggression and sexual restraint as that which preserves the self. Freud determined that ego instincts and the reality principle were also aspects of our primal nature, inherited from ancient ancestors (Freud, 1911). Spend too much of your time getting laid then you'll let your guard down, and with your pants down, your ass and the rest of you will be eaten by predators. Thanks, Jean Markale, for inviting us to move on from that primeval threat. Or, no thanks. We agree with Alexander (1989) that we still contend with predators, but they're not just in nature. They're embodied in our competition with one another, as the recreationally violent, or as critics and censors. At one societal pole are rapists and murderers. Halfway to the other: snake oil peddlers, sex and speech police. Also, Markale presumed the beneficent nature of women as he exhorted submission to "what they stand for." And the taboos besetting man and womankind seem relative. Father-daughter incest is a universal taboo, but society only began talking about it openly in the last century. Also, denial of widespread sexual abuse of women by men has yielded to openness only recently.[7]

What about mother-son or same-sex incest, or female-to-male sexual abuse? Bly (1990) offered a critique of the postfeminist era, tongue-tied, passive "soft male"; he warned against the possessiveness of mothers, but skirted the sexual implications. He may even have had secretive, object-substituting porn or sex addicts in mind when he wrote the following: "The soft male was able to say 'I can feel your pain, and I consider your life as important as mine, and I will take care of you and comfort you'. But he could not say what he wanted, and stick by it" (Bly, 1990, p. 4). What stills the tongue and blocks man from asserting what he wants? Fear of harming women with violence or desire? Or of harming them with separation or abandonment? This mythopoeic view suggests a conundrum. Bly's

7. Stemple and Meyer (2017) cull statistics from the Bureau of Justice and the Center for Disease Control, finding that men and women are equally likely to experience nonconsensual sex, with 35% of male victims reporting at least one female perpetrator. The criteria for sexual assault by women involve the concept of "made to penetrate" as a requirement for assault. With respect to incest, Osborne (2015) observed that our society views mothers as nurturers, idolizing and protecting motherhood. Holmes, Offen, and Waller (1997) also observed that men and boys are much less likely to report sexual abuse, perhaps reflecting tautological beliefs about femininity and victimization, though Kelly et al. (2002) conducted a study in which 17 of 67 men who endured sexual abuse during childhood also reported mother-son incest.

"soft male" observations of the 90s contrast with the "women have changed, but men haven't" views of Terrence Real (1998, 2003). Bly (1990) thought a significant number of postfeminist-era men had welcomed feminine consciousness, receiving feminine wisdom versus imparting masculine wisdom as patriarchs are inclined to do. But it wasn't really working. These men had burned draft cards while women burned bras and weren't harming the earth, but they were unhappy, Bly (1990) observed: they lacked resolve, decisiveness, and were unable to bring their natural "fierce" masculinity to relationships with women. Having lowered the sword, they had unwisely discarded it.

Today, feminists might not subscribe to the views of Markale or Bly, being more concerned with pragmatism than with history or mythology. Today, women may want men to sacrifice their lives or desires, to protect them from physical dangers or to perform physical jobs they either can't or don't want to do. And some of today's women share these burdens with men. Meanwhile, tall, muscular, crew-cut, rescuer-type men or even salty dogs remain preferable to many women who otherwise lament the pressure society places on *them* to achieve psychophysical ideals. The women of the baby boomer generation and milieu didn't know rap. They loved pop stars who emulated The Beatles ("I Wanna Hold Your Hand"), but also those who cloned Led Zeppelin ("I Wanna Give You Every Inch of My Love"). Lately, progressive gender politics indict the masculine gaze while admonishing women about the feminine swoon,[8] or their lust for *bad* men. Meanwhile, women want men to help raise children and be emotionally available; to have sex with attention to their partner's pleasure, not just their own.

If women presenting for treatment think their partners' sexuality wanton, we wonder the following: Did they think this before discovery? Do they think this of most men, not just sex addicts?

8. We might add to this admonishing trend the antecedent maternal "loom" described by Beebe (2016). Excess arousal is generated in an infant by a mother who moves too closely, or too much into an infant's face; this results in defensive self-regulating gestures (closed eyes, turning away, hands up), to which the mother "sobers," or repairs, with cooing, "flirtatious" behaviors that subsequently yield reconnection.

And do the men who sheepishly take part in treatment expect their wives and girlfriends to be monogamous? To listen to some, you might think that women—not patriarchs—had invented monogamy to contain the promiscuity of men. In modern times this may be true, or women may be more inclined toward monogamy, regardless of what patriarchs intend. Like therapist and author Esther Perel (2017), we think men and women expect too much of one another, to be *everything* to one another. They want neat segregation of qualities: sexy beast acts on the dance floor or in the bedroom, followed by wholesome and quiet efficiency elsewhere. No leaks. They might call this flexibility, those schooled in OR theory might call it whole-object relations, but it's neither. Such verbosity betrays the failure of splitting defenses, while honesty and humility hold promise for a whole self, allowing leaks through our embattled repression barriers with less damage. Good enough? Among our psychodynamic contemporaries, we notice that yesteryear theorists like D. W. Winnicott (1952, 1960) and Wilfred Bion (1961a,1961b) seem more popular than Sigmund Freud (1905, 1909, 1912, 1913, 1924) or Melanie Klein (1935, 1946). Let us retain mother-blaming and the abusive father shakedown, and add society or culture as an object of concern. Let's keep the wonders of reverie, but drop pansexual theories, death instinct theory, taboos, and phallocentric bias.[9] Let us be just-good-enough as parents and partners, transitioning gently from one attachment to the next, taking our teddy bears with us so that we might ever remember or discover our childhoods. Above all, let's pause the download on our Darth Vaders and those fair and foul witches of history.

---

9. This assignment of phallocentric bias to psychoanalysis seems to ignore the influence of Klein, who adhered to Freud's theories of death instinct and Oedipal complex, but placed the roots of both near the onset of life, not during a genital stage between ages three and five. This is significant because in her widely taught theory, the prototype for OR is the breast, not the phallus, which alters the nexus between objects and early development, which in turn might make better sense of misogyny, and especially concepts like "internalized misogyny" (the loved, hated, and feared early object is female for male and female infants). So, the crux is not so much who is in charge of society (patriarchy/superego), but rather who gave or denied food. Put another way, our aggression is not so much derived from who we fear castration from when young, but who we bit and chewed when even younger?

CASE ILLUSTRATION: JILL AND RAY

While some may believe that we are perverting the concept of intersectionality by not making requisite subscriptions, we believe the intersections between sex addiction concepts and wider social beliefs reflect provider and consumer biases, not society as a whole. This is illustrated by the case of Jill and Ray.

> When they first met me, Jill and Ray were ensconced in separate programs that featured supportive group activity and individual therapy. They presented for couples therapy feeling grounded within their support networks, but were still at odds with each other, and fought daily. Ray declared that he was sober from his bottom line or "inner circle" behaviors, which included use of pornography and prostitutes and masturbating to fantasy on a regular basis. Jill had discovered the former pattern of behavior a year earlier, after tracking Ray's search history on their computer. Jill (who was in her thirties) had married Ray (a fifty-year-old divorcee) two years earlier and now appeared to regret that life decision. The couple was childless, although he had two teenage children from a previous marriage. This was Jill's first marriage; she did not have any children, nor did she seem to want children, at least not with Ray. Sitting with them was a tense experience. They'd flank each other, rarely making eye contact, with Jill's eyes fixed uncertainly on me as Ray looked askance, sometimes grimacing. Her legs and feet shook incessantly, and her voice quavered. Ray's demeanor and delivery were slower and less pressured. An obese man, he'd squirm uncomfortably in his seat. Jill frequently opened sessions by firing salvos like: "I know now that I just can't trust him!" Ray would respond with languid confusion: "I don't know what she's talking about."
>
> Ray was a self-identified sex addict in recovery through SAA, and it was mutually agreed that Jill was a victim of his acting out. Ostensibly, he was the privileged figure in the relationship. He made the money. He was the one who had exercised license. He was the one in the power-up position. It didn't look or sound that way in my office, however. She would dominate their exchanges, speaking more quickly, interrupting him with sudden rebukes or piercing questions that derailed him whenever he spoke. In response, Ray would slump, then recline or tilt against the side of the patient

couch, looking like a chastened boy who couldn't keep up with adult conversation. My interventions aimed to create space for some proper communication, or at least a semblance of listening, between these two difficult people. The blunt disputes about whether he'd acted out in the fashion she suspected, based upon purportedly irrefutable clues, didn't get very far. The clues included text messages from unknown sources that Ray wouldn't (or couldn't) identify, scam email solicitations that he couldn't explain to her satisfaction, and charges on his credit card that betrayed suspicious locations that Ray had visited (which he dismissed as innocuous work excursions).

Jill was convinced that Ray was guilty of a slew of acting out behaviors not yet discovered, and I was failing in my role as walking polygraph by not eliciting the necessary confessions. Ray had, in fact, taken a polygraph a week before their first session with me—which he had passed. Jill rejected the results, claiming that the wrong questions had been asked, even though she had provided them herself in consultation with her first therapist. She declared that she knew better what to ask now, admitting to naiveté but demanding a second polygraph. Somewhat contrarily, she also suggested that Ray, with his gift for sneaking around, was capable of cheating the exam. "Not again," Ray balked, citing the cost (roughly $400 per test). He asked why he should take the test if Jill wouldn't accept results that didn't fit her preconceptions. (This was about the only cogent argument he managed to land.) Despite this standoff, Ray did agree to subsidize Jill's admission to a sex addict partner's treatment program: a two-week stint in a residential facility that provided psychoeducational groups and strategies to cope with symptoms of hyperarousal, dissociation, depression, and emotional reexperiencing. The couple agreed that she'd benefit from intensive support, after which she could return to individual and couples therapy, better able to self-soothe after highly stressful, "triggering" exchanges with Ray.

Ray naively hoped that, after bonding with similarly afflicted women, Jill would return calmer, ready to listen, and more trusting. I was skeptical, believing neither party was ready to think rather than act, and my skepticism was affirmed as Jill resumed couples sessions. She indeed seemed calmer, less pressured in her speech and less brittle in tone. But there was a sting in her calmer voice; a smooth air of entitlement had replaced her formerly frenetic anger.

I'd received a warning of sorts the day before the first return session when the director of her two-week program called to consult with me regarding her discharge plan. During a 10-minute exchange, this psychologist abruptly asserted that he'd fully assessed Jill's trauma syndrome, had conducted a telephone interview with Ray, and had decided that he was a sociopath and she was being terrorized by a systematic pattern of abuse. To substantiate these remarkable statements, he reeled off symptoms of her trauma and cited Jill's report that, just one week prior to admission for her two-week treatment (around the time of their last couples session with me), she had barricaded herself with furniture in her bedroom, frightened that an agitated and violent Ray was endangering her safety. "I think she needs someone to advocate for her and persuade him to move out of their home," the psychologist decreed, implying that the someone ought to be me.

I was taken aback, wondering how to challenge the perspective of this unctuous fellow professional. I agreed that Jill and Ray seemed ill-equipped to cope with the stressors of couples therapy. I asked about the details of his assessment and the stories he'd heard from Jill. Had there been a police report documenting the "terrorizing" incident he'd described? Had Jill suffered any injuries on this or any other occasion? (My prior assessment had not revealed a history of physical abuse.) And why hadn't they alerted me or their other therapists to this incident, or manifested the injuries that were purportedly incurred during the muddy time frame? I also asked the psychologist to share what had been said in Ray's telephone interview that demonstrated sociopathy. His patience wearing thin, the psychologist replied in a clipped voice that he believed Jill's story about the bedroom barricade. He also relayed her report that Ray had raped her numerous times by continuing to penetrate her when she was drunk and nearly passed out. During their telephone interview, Ray had denied the barricade event and memory of any nonconsensual sex with Jill, pointing out that they'd both been drunk on numerous occasions and were thus forgetful of event details, but the psychologist appeared to interpret these denials as proof of his sociopathy. I asked him to speculate why Jill, who had participated in therapy over three formats for over a year, had not mentioned anything about physical abuse to any other professional.

"I'm afraid I don't direct people to move out of their homes," I finally declared. (I wanted to add that I didn't work for him, but I held my tongue.) "I see," he replied tersely. His last tactic was to challenge my assessment skills. After reiterating his posttreatment recommendation, he suggested that therapists not specifically trained in his trauma model don't ask the right questions. He queried, in a rather dubious tone, whether I had asked them about nonconsensual sex. "No, but I did ask whether either party had ever had sex or experienced sex while unconscious." After attending a sexual abuse workshop many years ago, I make a point to ask this question if I know of—or sense—a disturbed sexual history. Jill and Ray did have a disturbed sexual history. In fact, their relationship had been the trigger for the breakup of Ray's first marriage. Jill had at least been in collusion with Ray's acting out during this period; they first met when she was working as a stripper in a gentleman's club.

"So, what'd they say?" asked the psychologist. I replied with the following: "*They* didn't. She reported that they'd once gotten drunk together, with Ray passing out just before they started having sex. Next, she felated him, attempting to revive Ray from his stupor, but failing. I'm paraphrasing. Not only did she not think that she had raped him, she actually thought she was fulfilling one of his fantasies, giving him a 'wet' dream. She characterized his passing out as an abandonment of her prior to the act of sex—thought he'd gotten sex elsewhere and was thus unavailable to her. Is that the kind of incident you were thinking about?" Pause. "You know it's not," the psychologist replied rancorously. For the record, I find that most collaborators are not so insistent about their approaches or assessments, which helps professionals examine their assumptions more openly. However, some in this niche field are fighting a cause, and they won't tolerate much fighting back, so collaboration with them really means recruitment into their conclusions and methods. To my apparent rival, I was merely an impudent, punching-above-my-pay-grade. At the end of our exchange, he declared that Jill and Ray needed a CSAT to help them, not me.

The acronym CSAT refers to Certified Sex Addiction Therapist, a credential earned through a limited liability company called the International Institute for Trauma and Addiction Professionals (IITAP). IITAP was established by Patrick Carnes, who is more or less credited with popularizing the term sex addiction and evangelizing its clinical validity alongside a posse of adherents. To become a CSAT you must complete about 20 days of training, be supervised by another CSAT for 30 hours, earn an additional 15 units of continuing education every 2 years, and pay a biannual fee. Incidentally, CSATs are not required to obtain advanced training in human sexuality and do not have to undergo an examination process to obtain their stamp of expertise. As a result of search engine dominance, CSAT members exert hegemony over sex addiction treatment and comprise the dominant readership of sex addiction literature; their perspective, in turn, informs what is disseminated on the subject of sex addiction. However, when you consider that requirements to become a Certified Drug and Alcohol Abuse Counselor include thousands of hours of direct contact experience plus hundreds of hours of education specific to substance use disorders to achieve certification, the CSAT credential seems, by comparison, rather slight.

There should have been a way for that specialist and me to pool our opinions and reconcile inconsistencies in the case of Jill and Ray. When I consider the assumptions beneath our exchange, I imagine that untangling them might have been messy. Without the late suggestion of violence or a slip that Ray may or may not have admitted to, would there still have been reason to ask Ray to leave because he wouldn't take another polygraph? What if Jill had admitted initiating either violence or sexual acting out, like the behavior reminiscent of Lot's daughters?[10] I suppose it might seem to some, echoing

10. From the Biblical book of Genesis: a reference to two virgin daughters who intoxicate their father, having sex with him without his knowledge, and subsequently giving birth to Moab and Ammon.

Nussbaum (1995), that Jill was perpetrating a benign act on that occasion, making a reasonable assumption of Ray's consent, but I think my psychologist colleague's biases revealed a paternalistic streak, and this is one area in which sex addiction specialists and patriarchs may be allies in their otherwise-not-intersecting beliefs. A progressively minded therapist would likely think that more economically privileged partners are best positioned to move out. A patriarch might think a separation unnecessary but, if pressed, might sanction the prescription because a man ought to protect his wife or at least provide for her materially.

Finally, what of my own biases? I considered whether the tidbit of knowledge that Jill had been a stripper had diminished my empathy for her, or rendered me skeptical of her assertions. I'd examined my countertransference on the matter, including my distrust of performance and performers, and my inclination toward judgment, except when it comes to justice. (I have never thought clinicians should take sides before there are facts or admissions.) For what it's worth, I did worry that Ray may have been the monster that Jill later claimed he was, and that her dysregulated presence in my office had manifested a trauma syndrome and not just an indignant attitude. I also wondered if her recall of the nonconsensual oral sex episode was selective. Could it have been an acted-out negation, reflecting a desire for the power-up position in contrast to the reality of their pairing? My neutral stance as a therapist didn't spare me the anxiety of not knowing. Was I wrong to not support her more directly? Regarding therapist desire: anxiety is a consequence of a quintessentially psychodynamic position—the desire to be neutral.

Ray continued to deny abusing Jill, sexually or otherwise, and remained wholly oblivious as to whether he'd been abused. Or, perhaps he was not so much oblivious as concealing, feeling as entitled to act out sexually as any patriarch of yesteryear, but patronizing Jill and—by extension—feminism by driving his true feelings underground; giving more abuse than he got but acting passively before witnesses; and preferring the old-school image of protector/sacrificial figure. He may have been manipulating everyone. I don't know, though I understand that pigs are smarter than dogs. In any case,

I deferred all conclusions, thinking the story had been thinly told with polemics skewed in favor of Jill, whose vehemently asserted victimhood soon leveraged habitation rights. Knowing that a resource-heavy Ray had options, I implied support of this resolution, asking Ray, "What happens if you stay?" He didn't have an answer, so he took the hint and packed his bags, which appeared to support one of my theories. Other, perhaps less urgent questions remained unanswered. Once, I asked about the original context of Jill and Ray's relationship: the affair they'd had together, which betrayed at least one other woman who barely got mentioned. Both were reticent on that subject, and I'm sure that observation further impacted my thinking as to the binary divides more readily assigned by my adversarial colleague: Who is the victim and who is the perpetrator? Who packs the overnight bag? Who leaves for the Arctic?

CHAPTER 3

Individual Therapy with the Sex Addict

In Rumi's poem, "On Resurrection Day," he says, "On Resurrection Day your body / testifies against you. / Your hand says, 'I stole money' / Your lips 'I said meanness' / Your feet 'I went where I shouldn't," and here comes part relevant to this book, "Your genitals 'Me too.'"

This poem by Rumi and translated by Barks (2004) speaks to the sense that one's body does not lie for us. It knows what has been done to it and what we have done with it. We may also consider this to be an example of what we refer to as unconscious or implicit mental process. We may have a sense of knowing that something happened to our body but not be able to remember it consciously.

The poem goes on to say, "They will make your praying / sound hypocritical. / Let the body's doing speak openly now, / without your saying a word, / As a student's walking behind a teacher / says, 'This one knows more clearly / than I the way.'" How many times do our patients try to explain away their actions with their words!

Let us not glorify the body as the supreme leader that always knows the best way to go. I think merely what is being conveyed in the second half of this poem is that our words may be hypocritical if what we say is disconnected from the wisdom of the body. The body should be listened to but not always obeyed. In psychodynamic approaches we are interested not only in what is not said but what happens in the body and in one's dreams and fantasies.

A Psychodynamic Approach

This chapter digs deeper into the psychodynamic approach. We, the authors, were both trained in the developmental, self, and OR approach of James F. Masterson, MD. Over the last two decades, this approach has been influenced significantly by advances in interpersonal neurobiology and attachment theory. We owe much of our thinking about how to conduct psychotherapy to Masterson, a strict, intelligent, thoughtful, and compassionate teacher.[1]

We refer to the people we work with as "patients." Many prefer the term "clients," feeling that this term assumes a more equal stature between the professional and those seeking their services. Our use of the term "patient" comes from two important experiences:

1. James Masterson came from a medical model and always referred to his clients as patients. Decades of work with his model have rubbed off and it feels awkward to use the term "client."
2. After some years working in a hospital setting, Joe has also become accustomed to the term "patients."

In using this word we are not attempting to elevate ourselves and diminish the patient. At the same time, the inequality in the relationship between professional and patient should be acknowledged. We do have something to offer the patient that the patient does not have. This is why they pay us. They believe we can be of help to them. Ignoring this inequality in the relationship can lead to harmful boundary violations.

We have a unique psychodynamic approach to the treatment of the sex addict and his family. Just like any other approach, it takes on the idiosyncrasies of the individual practitioner. One of the outstanding features of psychodynamic work is that the selfhood of the therapist is acknowledged and taken into account. The examination of transference and countertransference is fundamental to the psychodynamic approach. Our voice is influenced by our genetics and all of our experiences in life. Any work we do as therapists is largely about the unique personality and attachment style that we bring to the task. This cannot be understated. If we ignore the role of ourselves in the work, we do so at our own peril and to the detriment of the work. Both we and our patients will suffer.

---

1. On a personal note from Joe: At times he felt harsh, like when he was pressing me hard in supervision with a difficult patient. But most of the time I felt gratitude and appreciation toward him. He saw and understood me. He was a mentor and friend. Some of my favorite memories involve him.

In an important paper, Shedler (2010) shared the results of a comprehensive meta-analysis of the efficacy of different psychotherapeutic approaches. In particular, he noted that psychodynamic approaches are much more effective than believed by the clinical and lay community alike. According to Shedler, the psychodynamic approach includes the following elements:

Focus on affect and expression of emotion. This contrasts with approaches such as CBT, in which the focus is on thoughts and actions. The fact that a patient acted out (the behavior) is not as important as the feelings that were experienced before, during, and after the event. Thoughts are explored in the psychodynamic approach, but affect is believed to be a more powerful driver of behavior. We believe it is important to reflect on behavior also but not to the exclusion of feelings, thoughts, and fantasy.

Exploration of attempts to avoid distressing thoughts and feelings. Alternatively referred to as *defense analysis*, the therapist engages the patient in a discussion of the lengths to which the patient seems willing to go (such as sexual acting out with severe consequences) to avoid painful feelings.

Identification of recurring themes and patterns. Focusing on recurring themes is a good indicator of unconscious forces that may be at work in the person's psyche in which a person repeats an event or its circumstances over and over again in an apparent attempt to work through or achieve mastery over a past trauma or painful event.

Discussion of past experience (developmental focus). In contrast to behavioral approaches, which focus more on current disturbing behavior and thoughts than on the past, in psychodynamic approaches the attachment experience of the patient in childhood is viewed as laying important groundwork for future relationships. We see the past as extremely relevant, but not to the exclusion of the present.

Focus on interpersonal relations. The descriptions of interpersonal relations allow us to get a sense of the person. How does the patient describe his wife? His friends? How do they describe him?

A patient may be quite successful in his work, but how does he manage the intimate relationships in his life? This is where the narcissist, for example, is most vulnerable. He may be able to maintain an illusion of grandiosity before those who only know him casually, but to his family and intimates, he is exposed in a way that may be unbearable to him.

Focus on the therapy relationship. The relationship between patient and therapist and the feelings invoked in the therapist are clues to the intrapsychic life of the patient. Likewise, the feelings that the therapist invokes in the patient often reveal the nature of the early OR in the patient's life. Some of the most important therapeutic work takes place in the transference.

Exploration of fantasy life. Fantasy can be conscious or unconscious. An example of a conscious fantasy is when a patient describes their sexual fantasies in detail. Exploring such fantasies, which often play an important role in masturbation, can be helpful in exploring issues of sexual orientation. Unconscious fantasies may be revealed in a patient's dreams (Shedler, 2010, pp. 99–100).

Another element of psychodynamic psychotherapy we would add, but that didn't make Shedler's list, is **Exploration of unconscious process.** We would like to think that we are in control of our minds and that we make important life decisions on the basis of conscious, rational thoughts. Neuroscience assures us that nothing could be further from the truth. The majority of our motivations in day-to-day life are unconscious. When you walk into a crowded theater to select a seat, there are unconscious processes at play that assess risk and comfort. You are moved toward one seat and away from another based on the people who are already seated. When walking down the street talking on your cell phone, you may cross to the other side because your amygdala is activated by an approaching person who appears menacing. In a conversation, you may unconsciously steer away from one subject and toward another.

Think about a patient who writes a check to his therapist but forgets to sign it. This may lead to an exploration of previously unconscious anger toward the therapist. If the patient has felt deprived of a perceived need for instruction, he, in turn, deprives the therapist of payment. The idea of the unconscious was perhaps Freud's most important contribution to the field of psychotherapy. An experience in psychodynamic psychotherapy affords a patient the opportunity to delve into these areas of the unconscious to understand hidden motivations and self-sabotaging behavior.

Multiple sessions per week, which are common in psychodynamic psychotherapy, allow for a deepening of experience. By meeting with such frequency, a patient is less likely to focus on the news of the week or recounting of events. He is more likely to explore thoughts, feelings, and memories. As the therapeutic relationship develops and defenses are relaxed, the patient's focus shifts: he talks less about what happens *to* him and more of what happens *in* him.

Efficacy of Psychodynamic Approaches

Here's the conclusion of Shedler's (2010) meta-analysis on different approaches to the treatment of mental illness (including the use of pharmaceuticals):

> Empirical evidence supports the efficacy of psychodynamic therapy. Effect sizes for psychodynamic therapy are as large as those reported for other therapies that have been actively promoted as "empirically supported" and "evidence based." In addition, patients who receive psychodynamic therapy maintain therapeutic gains and appear to continue to improve after treatment ends. (Shedler, 2010, p. 98)

Much of the work on and improvements in patients' lives take place after the termination of therapy. The process of integrating the gains of psychodynamic psychotherapy takes place as life unfolds and as patients consult the internalized representation of their therapists. It's as if the therapist continues to live within them as a source of comfort, guidance, and ongoing admonitions to pay attention to feelings and the attempts to defend against them. When patients can find no compassion for themselves, they can remember the compassion their therapists showed toward them.

Many of our patients enter therapy with the goal of feeling better. Because human nature leads us to eliminate suffering whenever we can, it may seem counterintuitive to let patients dip into painful affects or experience vulnerable states of mind that threaten their sense of self-worth or challenge their ego ideal. If it were possible to leapfrog these affects and arrive in a better place, most people would sign up without hesitation. Masterson often warned his students about caring too much about making their patients feel better. He believed that *getting* better and *feeling* better were two different things. This was a refrain often heard by his students. He believed that if you suffer from a personality disorder, you must first feel worse to get better. This is because the patient is rewarded for regression by the internalized objects. And defensive merger with the other likewise feels good but the healthy response, differentiation, feels bad. If a patient perseveres, he arrives at the best of all worlds: he gets better and actually feels better about getting better.

The first time a patient considers the idea that pain must indeed precede gain, it may not make a lot of sense rationally, but there is a feeling of truth about it. To live in a fantasy world or a state of denial may feel better, but it usually leads to pain and dysfunction for the individual and those around him. Facing himself honestly may be quite painful, but eventually it can lead to living a more truthful and honest life. To paraphrase a friend, "The truth may set you free but first it's going to piss you off."

In his poem "Warning to the Reader," Robert Bly (1992) describes how blackbirds get caught in empty grain silos. They attempt to free themselves by flying up to the cracks between the boards where a little light enters, but end up as skeletons on the floorboards. The key to getting out is not via the upward trajectory, but down low through the subterranean holes where the rats enter. However, blackbirds don't like going underground. Similarly, our patients come in wanting to fly up toward the light. They believe if only we would share with them the secrets of the solution they could easily escape peril. It's often disappointing for them to hear us say, "I don't have a quick solution. I think this is going to take some time and it will probably be quite difficult."

The goal of therapy is to help the patient gain access to their real *self*, a concept central to Masterson's model. People often equate the real self with D. W. Winnicott's (1965) idea of the *true self*, a concept that honors Freud. According to Winnicott (1965), Freud divided the self into "a part that is central and powered by the instincts (or by what Freud called sexuality, pregenital and genital), and a part that is turned outwards and is related to the world" (p. 140). The central part is the true self and the outward part is the false self. To Winnicott (1965), the function of the *false self* is to "hide and protect the true self" (p. 142). He goes on to say, "In health: the False Self is represented by the whole organization of the polite and mannered social attitude, a 'not wearing the heart on the sleeve', as might be said. Much has gone to the individual's ability to forgo omnipotence and the primary process in general, the gain being the place in society which can never be attained or maintained by the True Self alone" (Winnicott, 1965, p. 143). In contrast, Masterson's concept of *real self* includes the reality requirements of the external world. The individual must negotiate between the needs of the society and the self to come up with a successful compromise; the successful results of this compromise are the following capacities of the real self (Masterson, 2000):

Spontaneity and aliveness of affect. The ability to experience affect deeply with liveliness, joy, vigor, excitement, and spontaneity.

Self-entitlement. From early experiences of mastery, coupled with parental acknowledgment and support of the emerging self, the sense that the self is entitled to appropriate experiences of mastery and pleasure as well as the environmental input necessary to achieve them. Self-entitlement is deficient in the borderline patient and excessive in the narcissist.

Self-activation, self-assertion, and self-support. The identification of unique individuated wishes, the use of autonomous initiative and assertion to express them in reality, and the ability to support and defend them when under attack.

Acknowledgment of self-activation and maintenance of self-esteem. Recognition that the self has dealt with an affective experience or an environmental issue or task in a positive, adaptive manner. This is the vehicle for autonomously fueling adequate self-esteem. Patients without this capacity don't recognize when they have taken steps in support of the real self. For example, a patient may recall a forgotten traumatic event and relay it coherently, then devalue their effort by saying something like, "I feel like I'm rambling now."

Soothing of painful affects. The ability to devise means to limit, minimize, and soothe painful affects. A patient with an underdeveloped soothing capacity may compensate for it by acting out in an addictive manner. The pain is soothed temporarily but it returns later because the patient has not learned more adaptive ways to soothe it.

Continuity of the self. The acknowledgment that the "I" of one experience is continuous over time and related to the "I" of another experience. The real self adapts to the needs of the moment and expresses itself differently in different contexts.

Commitment. The ability to commit the self to an objective or a relationship and to persevere, despite obstacles, to attain that goal or maintain that relationship.

Creativity. The use of the self to take old familiar patterns and change them into new, unique, and different patterns. According to Masterson, the emergence of creativity in a patient's life is a hallmark of successful treatment for a person with a disorder of the self.

Intimacy. Expression of the self fully in a close relationship with minimal anxiety about abandonment or engulfment (for the borderline patient), exposure of inadequacy (for the narcissist), or fear of being enslaved or controlled by the other (for the schizoid patient).

Autonomy. The ability of the self to regulate its affect and its socioemotional relationships in the absence of an empathic other.

Along these lines, sexual addiction or sexual acting out is viewed as a defense against the real self and the real self affects. But the affects of the real self are often experienced as the blackbird experiences the subterranean rat hole. They are perceived as perilous. A patient once shared, "Sometimes I feel really bad about myself but when I make love to a beautiful woman it is the most effective antidepressant I have ever known. It's so much easier than addressing why I feel bad about myself. Easier than exercising and eating right . . . at least in the short term." As therapists, we can facilitate thinking, feeling, and authentic expression of the real self by first establishing a therapeutic alliance. We listen deeply to what the patient is saying and don't utilize standardized treatment protocols. We put the patient—not a manual—first. The British analyst Wilfred Bion (1967) urged therapists to approach each session without memory or desire (i.e., without a manual):

> The psychoanalyst should aim at achieving a state of mind so that at every session he feels he has not seen the patient before. If he feels he has, he is treating the wrong patient. This procedure is extremely penetrating. Therefore the psychoanalyst must aim at a steady **exclusion of memory and desire** and not be too disturbed if the results appear alarming at first. He will become used to it and he will have the consolation of building his psychoanalytic technique on a firm basis of intuiting evolution and NOT on the shifting sand of slight experience imperfectly remembered which rapidly gives way not to experience, but to neurologically certain decay of mental faculty. (p. 2)

Although it is not the popular choice for treating sex addicts, we feel that psychodynamic psychotherapy is an important and effective approach that has been overlooked in the literature. Most practitioners who work with sexual addiction use models more akin to CBT. There is a general belief held by our colleagues that CBT is more effective. However, Shedler (2010) concluded that, "No research findings ever suggested that manualized CBT was more effective than psychodynamic therapy. It was just more often researched" (p. 1). We have noticed something interesting about CBT over the years of working with CBT therapists. When practitioners of CBT seek out their own individual therapy, they usually pick a psychodynamic therapist.[2]

We're not sure what to make of this phenomenon. When psychodynamic therapists seek therapy on the other hand, they usually choose a psychodynamic therapist. Someday we will ask a CBT therapist about this. If you are one of those, send us a note. We'd love to hear your thoughts.

---

2. Joe remembers attending a conference with a well-known CBT couples therapist. It was a large meeting and at the morning break he was overheard talking about his "current analyst." He was comparing him to "his last analyst."

As the therapist listens there is a focus not only on what is said but what is not said. What is unconscious? Consider this interaction with a female sex addict.

CASE ILLUSTRATION: SANDY

I returned from a one-week vacation and had this interaction with Sandy, one of my female sex addict patients. Before I left for vacation, she had broken up with Corey and sworn that she would never go back to him.

Sandy started, "Corey contacted me after the restraining order expired. We had a good talk. He said he still loves me and wants to be with me."

There is a significant pause where Sandy seems to be waiting for some response from me. It is almost as if she is expecting me to chastise her for talking to the man she had a restraining order against and who had, many times before, broken her heart like no one else. I remain silent, but curious.

Sandy continued, "We actually had sex . . . three times since I saw you last."

Another pause and a minute of silence. She is reporting what took place but not describing how this change of events has impacted her or how she made the decision to sleep with him. Again, she seems to be expecting to be chastised by me.

Therapist: And how is that for you?

Sandy: The sex was very good. Sex is always good between us. It always has been, even in the beginning. It's not like fucking but more like making love. My body responds to him very well and he is a kind and generous lover. It's always satisfying for me. On occasion we would have a quickie but mostly we are both satisfied with sex. Both of us climax.

Therapist: Yes, I think I recall you telling me once before that you two are very compatible sexually. I guess when I asked "how is this for you?" I was wondering how it feels for you to have reconnected with Corey after the breakup.

I am attempting to establish with Sandy that I will not be suggesting that she get back with Corey or break up with him. This is the definition of *therapeutic neutrality*. It's not my job to remind her that he is an alcoholic or that he took advantage of her or that he injured her when he grabbed her arm during an argument. She knows all these things and probably expects me to object to this recent news of a reunion. She will have to make her own decision (or non-decision) about what to do with Corey. I simply ask about her feelings about having him back in her life. At our next session:

Sandy: He was cheating on me within days of us having sex. I drove by the bitch's house the other day and his car was there. I can't believe anything he says. It's all lies and I fall for it every time. He can have me but he chooses this blonde party girl slut with the fake boobs that is ten years younger than him. He just doesn't want to grow up. He's like a teenager. All he wants to do is party and get high.

Revisiting the Definition of Sex Addiction

Alternatives to the term sex addiction include *sexual compulsivity* (defined in Chapter 1 as an "insistent, repetitive, unwanted urge to perform specific acts often in ritualized or routinized fashions" [Kalichman and Rompa, 1995]), "sexual acting out," or problem sexual behaviors. As noted in Chapter 2, patients tend to be white males, but as the case of Sandy illustrates, it should not be inferred that only white males are sex addicts. This just happens to best characterize the populations in our private practices. Female sex addicts are rare, but generally report seeking emotional intimacy though the vehicle of sex rather than anonymous sex by itself. To be fair, some men have a similar motive, but they may not be able to identify it as easily. Here's a definition of sex addiction.

> Sexual addiction involves the core elements of addiction: a craving state prior to behavioral engagement, or a compulsive engagement; an impaired control over behavioral engagement; and continued behavioral engagement despite negative consequences. (Potenza, 2006, p. 60)

There are complications with this rather simple definition. Imagine a patient who has never cheated before but starts an affair. What about a married person for whom masturbation interferes in the sexual relationship with a spouse because there is less desire for intercourse? Strictly speaking, both these individuals meet the criteria for sex addiction that we have just laid out. However, many professionals in the sex addiction treatment community would hesitate to label either of them a sex addict. Since DSM-5 did not rescue us from the ambiguity of the term by defining it for us, we are left to our own devices. We may prefer to speak of these two individuals as having sexual problems rather than as having sexual addiction.

Patients Mandated for Treatment

There is a major difference between a private practice and an agency like the ITC in northern California. Most therapists generally don't see court-mandated patients in a private practice setting. At ITC, a small minority of patients have been mandated for treatment. These patients, who are involved in the justice system, have had a judge order them to seek out or continue treatment. They may have been convicted of offenses such as possession or distribution of child pornography or sex with a minor. Some may have been caught in a sting operation in which the FBI posed as an underage minor and arrangements were made online to meet and have sex. Others may be awaiting trial and anticipating a mandate for treatment, or have been sentenced, served their time in jail, and are now on parole. Still others may be in a diversion program, in which they agreed to seek treatment in place of prosecution. Patients may be registered as sex offenders for the rest of their lives, allowing their neighbors and anyone in the general public to log onto Megan's Law website (www.meganslaw.ca.gov) and see their known aliases, photo, address, sex, height, weight, eye color, hair color, ethnicity, offense, and risk assessment.[3] To be listed as a sex offender is to be branded with the modern-day equivalent of a scarlet letter.

Legal Issues

In 2014, California passed a law that may have devastating effects on patients who are voluntarily seeking help for sexual addiction problems. Assembly Bill 1775 expanded the scope of the California child abuse reporting law sponsored by the CAMFT, requiring therapists to report any of their patients who have looked at child pornography online. The text of the law follows:

---

3. From Joe: Within a two-mile radius of my home there are 17 registered sex offenders. All are male. Fifteen are white and two are Hispanic. If I expand the search, I will find the occasional female.

> Under the act, sexual exploitation refers to, among other things, a person who depicts a child in, or who knowingly develops, duplicates, prints, or exchanges, a film, photograph, videotape, negative, or slide in which a child is engaged in an act of obscene sexual conduct, except as specified. Failure to report known or suspected instances of child abuse, including sexual abuse, under the act is a misdemeanor. . . . This bill . . . provide(s) that sexual exploitation also includes a person who knowingly downloads, streams, or accesses through any electronic or digital media, a film, photograph, videotape, video recording, negative, or slide in which a child is engaged in an act of obscene sexual conduct. (Child Abuse and Sexual Assault Act)

This law has already had a chilling effect on what patients are willing to discuss with their therapists (Mathews, 2019). Patients who view child pornography are hesitant to discuss their ego-dystonic behavior if they know they must be reported. One unintended consequence of this law is requiring a therapist to report a teenage patient who has been texting sexually explicit photos of themself to their boyfriend or girlfriend. Such activity, called sexting, is a fairly common practice among teenagers. A recent study (Madigan, 2018) that looked at over 100,000 teenagers between ages 12 and 17 years found that 14.8% had sent a sext and 27.4% had received a sext. Imagine a teenager being forced to register as a sex offender for life because they sent or received an explicit photo to or from their boyfriend or girlfriend. In *Mathews et al v Harris AB1775*, Don Mathews[4] is currently challenging the changes to the reporting law. After many appeals, the California Supreme Court agreed to hear the case and decide if mandating therapists to notify authorities that their patients are viewing child pornography violates those patients' rights to privacy. The state supreme refused to uphold the law and sent it back to the lower courts for trial. We think this is an important issue and support Mathews and his colleagues in their efforts to defeat this law because it undermines confidentiality, which is the foundation of treatment. If this challenge fails and other states follow California's lead, it may undermine the

4. Don Mathews is also the owner of the ITC in Walnut Creek, California.

process and limit the efficacy of the treatment of sex addicts in the United States in very significant ways.

Standardized Treatment Models

Before we get into the treatment of the sex addict, we'd like to comment on standardized treatment models. When someone touts the benefits of a particular treatment model and uses research to back up their claim, they are usually referring to an approach that has been "manualized" or standardized. In other words, a manual has been developed in an attempt to guide the therapist and make sure they are actually providing that type of therapy. There are practical problems here. Therapists are not identical copies of one another. There will be differences in the work of two therapists, even if they are working from the same manual. Also, just because a therapist is using the manual doesn't mean they are good at it. Aaron T. Beck was quoted in a *New York Times* article as saying, "You can't do cognitive therapy from a manual any more than you can do surgery from a manual" (Carey, 2004). For example, just because a therapist claims to use the approach taught by Patrick Carnes (a pioneer in the field of sex addiction treatment), it doesn't mean they are any good. The other problem with standardized treatments is that treatment model A doesn't necessarily work any better than treatment model B. In fact, Duncan (2005) demonstrated that:

> The preponderance of the data therefore indicates a lack of specific effects and refutes any claim of superiority when two or more bona fide treatments fully intended to be therapeutic are compared. If no specific technical operations can be reliably shown to produce a specific effect, then manualizing psychotherapy seems to make little sense. (p. 142)

We are belaboring this point to inoculate clinicians against the frequent claims that are made in print, in discussions with colleagues, and on glossy flyers that arrive at your office advertising a new how-to book or a workshop on the latest "evidence-based" treatment model. By the way, for an approach to be "effective" it must only show improvement over no treatment at all. The evidence comes from studies in which the improvement of the treatment group is compared to improvement in the no-treatment group. If the treatment group shows any significant improvement, the approach is deemed effective. Are we suggesting that you should not attend the conference that is advertised on that glossy flyer? Or that you were mistaken to purchase this book or any other book about psychotherapy? Absolutely not. Like you, we find new insights with every book we read and every conference we attend, and those insights eventually show up in the consulting room.

Our subjective experiences tell us that these changes in our approach are helpful to our patients. We are just suggesting that knowledge about the approach being used, along with a little humility, is not a bad thing. We are humbled quite regularly in our clinical work. Sometimes we may be absolutely certain that we know exactly what led to a patient's improvement throughout psychotherapy, then become sheepish when the patient describes to us in their own words what they thought was most helpful because it often has nothing whatsoever to do with what we imagined. Embarrassingly, sometimes patients repeat what they heard us say to them during a pivotal session two years earlier, and we are absolutely certain we said nothing of the sort! We believe that an essential element of healing in psychotherapy is the therapeutic relationship itself. It probably doesn't matter what we actually said to that patient two years ago. Something about our relationship has been healing for them, and perhaps even for us.

Discovery

discover **verb** *dis·cov·er* | \ *di-ˈskə-vər*
The process of finding, realizing, or unearthing something
(www.vocabulary.com)

Imagine that you arrive for your early morning dental appointment and a staff meeting has just concluded. An unfamiliar receptionist is managing the front desk on her own (there are normally two). When a dental assistant—who you have known for years—comes to get you, she is friendly but a bit reserved. Something in her face reveals that she is preoccupied. You're guided into the procedure room and as you sit in the dental chair you become aware of a slight uneasiness. Although you genuinely hate going to the dentist, you don't think it's about the procedure you're about to undergo. There is a strange feeling in the air suggesting to you that all is not well. Something is off. You feel as though you have discovered something in the social fabric of the workplace that is trying to stay hidden. Business as usual. Nothing to see here.

The assistant prepares you for the procedure and you engage in small talk about the weather. Then the dentist comes in. He also seems preoccupied. As you start to feel the effects of the nitrous oxide, you wonder if it is making you more sensitive to the emotional tone in the voices and movements of those around you. The procedure begins, and the dentist and assistant work together, but without their normal ease and efficiency. It's a bit clunky today. They don't flow with each other. He steps out of the room for a moment, and you hear him snap at a staff member. You ask the assistant if everything is alright. "Oh, yes, everything is wonderful," she responds in a higher-than-normal pitch. You sense that everything is *not* wonderful. The dentist comes back and finishes the long procedure. As you get ready to leave, you start to question yourself. Are you being too sensitive? Why do you need to dramatize the experience and imagine that something not so nice is going on underneath the surface? As therapists, we have learned to listen to our intuition and be curious about such feelings. Perhaps the phrase, "trust but verify" made popular by Ronald Reagan during the Cold War is a useful guide for therapists when we sniff out something that feels off, like that glass of milk a month past its expiration date. Was it the nitrous oxide or was your intuition telling you something? As you gather your coat and prepare to leave the office you hear one staff member talk to another about the events of yesterday, when the two receptionists from the front office quit on the spot without notice. Your perceptions are validated, and you are no longer questioning yourself. Now imagine you experience this situation in a relationship with a romantic partner.

On many occasions in the consulting room, a woman says, "I just have a feeling that something is wrong. He's not acting like himself. He seems different." Or, "I can't put my finger on it, but it seems like something is going on." A patient recently described looking at her husband's photos on his phone and wondering who the baby in the photo was. It turned out to be her husband's child, a product of an affair she knew about a few years before.

A wife described her husband wanting to try something new while making love: "It was so unlike him, he's never been interested in that kind of thing before . . . where did that come from?"

Another wife described how her husband looked alarmed after receiving a text message and immediately stashed his phone in his pocket; when she asked him who it was it took an extra second or two for him to answer. Sometimes the intuition that something is wrong sends a wife (or a husband) looking for clues to confirm the feeling. The next time he leaves his cell phone on the table and a text message comes in she might look to see who it's from. She may check his emails and discover with horror that he has been carrying on an illicit affair or at least acting with another in a way that is sure to lead to one. Or she may look at the browser history on his computer and discover that he has been visiting pornographic websites or advertisements for sex workers.

On the other hand, she may find nothing. She may begin to question her intuition and wonder if the feeling is more about her than her partner, or she may be haunted by the feeling for years without any validation. She may never mention it. She may begin to think that she is losing her mind. One woman received a desperate, angry call from her husband's lover after he tried to end a three-year-long affair, providing many painful details. One man, after walking in on his wife and her lover in his own bed, took the mattress out into the front yard and torched it. A married couple with an open relationship in which they frequently have sex with other couples or individuals have a strict policy that sex with others needs to be discussed between them before it happens; the husband brought them both to therapy when he discovered that she had sex with a friend without telling him.

When something is found out, it can set in motion a series of events that eventually lead to a phone call from a wife or girlfriend who wants her partner to attend individual or couples therapy. Sometimes discovery takes place during couples therapy. The couple may enter therapy to improve their relationship only to discover that without honesty it is difficult to have true intimacy. She might finally disclose a current affair or one that took place many years ago and is now over.

> With one recent individual therapy client, discovery was the result of a very conscious, deliberate process. The patient's affair resulted in pregnancy and his paramour decided to have the child. When reality and life circumstances required him to decide what action to take, he chose to stay with his wife and try to heal their

relationship. Eventually, in couples therapy, he told his wife about the affair and pregnancy. Only after two very difficult years of couples therapy and individual therapy was the new child slowly and successfully integrated into his family with his wife and teenage children.

Sometimes discovery begins with the seemingly innocuous comment of an individual therapist. In the midst of a patient describing a sharp decline in their sexual frequency and the apparent emotional unavailability of his wife, the therapist might wonder out loud, "Do you think she might be having an affair?" Even if she isn't, the husband can now think of nothing else. Maybe he becomes self-critical about his ignorance because he never thought about that himself. Maybe he secretly fears it and his therapist's utterance gives him permission to speak and explore the fear. Or maybe the therapist's suspicion alone, which may be based on the therapist's personal past, reifies the concern, moving the patient into a state of certainty. A dreadful certainty is sometimes easier to deal with than confusion and uncertainty. It's always preferable for the idea that "my partner may be having an affair" to come from the patient, *not* the therapist. If the affair is a nagging question in your mind, we suggest some self-reflection: Is this about your experience or the patient's experience? If it seems to be on the patient's mind, either consciously or unconsciously, ask yourself, "Why can't my patient consider this possibility? What is blocking them?"

Developing a Therapeutic Alliance

A *therapeutic alliance* can be defined as a mutual understanding that the patient and therapist are working together for the benefit of the patient in achieving the patient's stated goals. The patient's job is to show up on time, focus on themselves, and pay their bill. During sessions it is their responsibility to attempt to be as open as possible in discussing their problems, thoughts, and feelings with the therapist. The therapist's role is to listen intently to what is being said and not said, and to ask clarifying questions in an attempt to gain an understanding of the problem. As the therapist gains an understanding of the defenses being utilized by the patient, the therapist may interpret them to the patient or confront the patient with any self-destructive aspects. The therapist's feelings and internal responses to the patient are used to gain insight into the patients intrapsychic structure.

> When dissociated emotions are experienced by sensitive therapists, our bodies function like resonant tuning forks. (Stone, 2006, described in Marks-Tarlow, 2014, p. 81)

A psychiatrist colleague described his own tuning fork. When he has the urge to yawn during a session, he has come to trust that it is his personal and physiological response to a patient who is repressing anger, so he finds it useful to inquire about anger at such times. The colleague has found this to be a very effective, reliable tool to use during his patient sessions.

The client takes a risk in opening up to the therapist. As the therapist begins to understand the patient's experience, the therapist conveys that understanding to the patient, and trust begins to develop. As trust is developed, the patient gradually becomes willing to suspend his normal defenses and gains more access to the impaired real self. When the therapist is not attuned to the patient, the usual result for the patient is shame. On the other hand, attunement between them encourages and reinforces the patient's vulnerability. Without patient vulnerability, there can be little progress. This process establishes a therapeutic relationship in which the patient comes to trust that the therapist has his best interests at heart.

With mandated patients, trust is much harder to come by. A very clearly defined Release of Information agreement may be the first tool used to establish trust. In it, the patient can see that the therapist won't reveal his secrets to the court but will simply verify that he is attending his sessions and making a sincere effort in treatment. The patient begins to relax, seeing a major shift from therapy as an instrument of the justice system that gathers secret information to an opportunity to address his own needs. The therapist can help with his first goal, to get the justice system off his back and out of his personal life. The patient's sincere effort to reveal himself in therapy is rewarded.

Therapeutic Neutrality

We advocate a client-centered approach based on therapeutic neutrality. The patient—not the therapist—is at center stage. The therapist's role is not to set the agenda of treatment or educate or advocate any particular action. The therapist may make a suggestion to the patient, but this should be the exception rather than the rule. The job of the therapist is to listen intently, both to what the patient is saying and what he is not saying. It's not our job to help the patient move in the right direction. Instead, therapeutic neutrality involves helping him face down the defenses served by the sexual acting out (or the denial of it) and to understand what he has protected himself against: fears of intimacy, engulfment, exposure, and depression. Because patients are often acting out the desire to meet unconscious and unspoken relational needs (Director, 2002), awareness facilitates changes in behavior aimed at meeting those needs in a less destructive way. Exploring the fear of being seen accurately by the therapist and eventually by a partner may pave the way for more healthy risk-taking and emotional sharing in the relationship.

States of Mind

One of the neurological concepts that can facilitate our understanding of the patient and the best way to intervene is the concept of states of mind. Dan Siegel (2012) defined a state of mind as: "the total pattern of activations in the brain at a particular moment in time." This broadens the generally understood notion of a state of mind, typically considered to be the particular thoughts a person is having at any given moment. The broader definition considers not only thoughts but feelings, body sensations, interception cues, smells, sounds, memories, heart rate, and stomach distress. So when we talk about the state of mind that preceded a patient's phone call to a prostitute to set up an appointment, we are talking not just about the thoughts and fantasies of exciting sex, but also about the accelerated heartbeat, the sweating palms, the feeling of being desired, and even the awareness that such a feeling may be false. If a sex worker is familiar to the patient, the anticipatory state of mind may include the smell of her perfume and her hair, the feeling of holding her body in his arms, the tone of her voice, and an image of the hotel room where they last met.

Implicit Memory

Although it may seem counterintuitive, implicit memory, also called unconscious memory, is another useful concept in the consideration of psychodynamic treatment. Implicit memories are memories that we don't actually experience as memories. Conscious recall of a memory, like remembering a trip to the zoo as a child, is explicit memory. Say that you are watching a nature show on television and a close-up of an ostrich head startles you and makes your heart rate increase and your palms become sweaty. This may be an implicit memory based on an experience when you were riding through a wildlife park and an ostrich stuck its head through the open car window and attacked your head. Even if you don't remember the original event (you were only three years old, after all), your body remembers it and reacts accordingly. Say that an older sibling is watching the show with you and says, "Do you remember the time we went to that wild animal park and that ostrich started pecking on your head?" As you ask for more details and learn more about the event, it gives meaning to your bodily response. The implicit memory becomes explicit autobiographical memory, and you have made sense of the bodily experience and put it into context.

Procedural Memory

Procedural memory is a type of implicit memory (Lyons-Ruth, 2009). We remember how to do something (i.e., the procedure involved) but don't have the experience of remembering anything. Take riding a bike. You may not have hopped on one in many years, but once you do your body remembers how to maintain balance, pedal, brake, and steer. Riding a bike is a very complicated, precise body memory. To give you an appreciation for the capacities of the human mind, know that it's very difficult to teach a robot how to ride a bike.

Similarly, we have procedural memory of how to act around people in different types of situations. If someone is angry and raising their voice, a patient may find himself fading away and trying to hide or become small, a childhood survival strategy when Dad was drunk and having a rage episode. When his wife is enraged, he doesn't realize he is remembering anything, but may find himself responding similarly as he responded to his father at those moments. What is absent is the experience of saying to himself, "I am remembering something now." It can be very useful to make such memories explicit and sort out these experiences during therapy.

In 2018, when the national news carried a story of how Attorney General Jeff Sessions used his authority to prosecute websites that advertised prostitution[5] and showed photos of some homepages on air, one of my patients was *triggered* (he had an implicit procedural memory recall). After seeing the familiar website, he contacted a sex worker later that night and set up an appointment, telling his wife he had to go into the office. He had been sober for nine months and didn't even recognize what the trigger was until he discussed it in therapy three days later. The image triggered his memory of the procedure of contacting a sex worker, and he picked up his phone to search for the phone number of the woman he hadn't had sex with for nine months.

We've all heard similar stories about the alcoholic who walks past his favorite liquor store and finds himself buying a bottle of whiskey after five years of sobriety. Or the drug addict, in recovery for 10 years, who runs into his dealer when he is out of town and uses for the first time in a decade.

CASE ILLUSTRATION: TONY

Tony, a 48-year-old married surgeon and father of four, was referred to me for individual therapy from a sex addiction treatment program. At our first meeting I was struck by his physical presence. Tony is a very large and intimidating man. He is about 6 feet, 5 inches, probably weighs about 270 pounds, and is extremely muscular and lean. The voicemail he had left for me was somewhat pleading, requesting that I call him back soon because he was "white knuckling it." This term is often used in 12-step programs to describe an addict who is not working on his recovery but is abstinent by sheer force of will. It implies that relapse is close by. During our first meeting he explained that he is a recovering cocaine addict and alcoholic, and self-identifies as a sex addict.

A brief history revealed that he found his father's pornography collection when he was seven years old. As he got older, Tony used to masturbate to the images he found in his father's stash.

5. Justice Department Leads Effort to Seize Backpage.Com, the Internet's Leading Forum for Prostitution Ads, and Obtains 93-Count Federal Indictment. Monday, April 9, 2018, www.justice.gov.

He showed them to a neighborhood boy, and eventually they would masturbate together. On occasion, he asked the other boy to touch his penis and he'd become aroused. This pattern continued into adulthood as he sought out other males to masturbate with him or for him. Sometimes he receives oral sex from them. He meets these men at gay bars, bathhouses, or nude beaches. Occasionally he hooks up on Grindr, a sexual hookup site for gay and bisexual individuals that he can access on his phone. He never provides oral sex for these men but hopes to receive it himself. He carries a wig to the hookups and asks the other man to wear it. Sometimes the other man refuses, but they have sex anyway.

Putting another man's penis in his mouth would be too disgusting for him and the mere thought of it makes him feel nauseous. Having a man on his knees in front of him makes him feel like his penis is being worshiped. He's proud of the size and shape of his penis and is quite stimulated by other's appreciation of it as well. Tony identifies as heterosexual but is frustrated that his wife doesn't have the same level of sexual desire as he does. He is offended by the suggestion (from one of the men he has acted out with) that he is gay or bisexual. If she was willing, he would like to have sex several times a day with his wife. He views his acting out with other men as purely a way to satisfy his sexual desire. He rationalizes that it doesn't threaten his marriage because he doesn't act out with other women. To him this seems reasonable, and he was quite surprised at his wife's anger when he confessed to her during intercourse that he likes to receive oral sex from men. He told me that he found it very arousing to share this with her.

Early in his career, during his fourth year of medical school, Tony was hospitalized twice for cocaine addiction and completed two 30-day treatment programs. The treatments were mandated by the hospital and medical school when a colleague caught him using cocaine in the doctor's lounge at work. After his second inpatient treatment, he finally got clean by attending regular NA meetings. The only other treatment he received was treatment for sexual addiction at a local clinic where he participates in group therapy on an ongoing basis.

Tony is the younger of two sons. His older brother seems to be favored by the parents because he was a more obedient child and avoided the problems Tony had. Tony's father is a well-known heart surgeon who was fired from the local hospital where he worked. Tony realized later in life that the firing was caused by his sexual relationships with multiple female coworkers and at least one sexual harassment claim. Tony's mother is a journalism professor at a local university. He remembers his mother's disgust at his father's infidelity. To Tony, she seemed to see all men in the same way, as filthy pigs. He remembers her as cold and aloof and can't recall any memories of her being affectionate or expressing love toward him. She was smart, cool, and detached.

Tony has very few memories of elementary school. He was awkward in middle school because he was sexually mature before the other boys in his class. He had facial hair in eighth grade and had to shave every day. He was popular in high school because he was a good football player, but he was "afraid" of girls. He didn't date until college, where he always seemed to get good grades without too much effort. He played football at a top-tier college and studied premed. He drank and experimented with drugs in college but was serious about football so his drug use never became problematic. He had a significant knee injury his senior year and had to sit out most of the season. He had hoped to play professional football, but after missing most of his senior season his father convinced him to take the MCATs (Medical College Admissions Tests) and apply to medical school. He took up cocaine in medical school to stay awake during the long hours required for study and internships. Tony is a recovering cocaine addict in a stable recovery and has not used for 14 years. He attends Cocaine Anonymous (CA) and NA meetings about five to seven times each year. No one in either program has been willing to sponsor him in the long term because they say the frequency of his attendance is insufficient.

He has narcissistic defenses but they are not sufficient to meet the criteria for Narcissistic Personality Disorder. He does not have a mood or anxiety disorder and takes no prescribed psychiatric medicines. He does have CSBD and continues to act out sexually despite negative consequences in his life, such as intense shame, marital problems, and financial and occupational problems related to absences or tardiness at work.

Therapeutic Frame

Arriving on time for therapy, paying on time, starting and ending the sessions on time, and having a clear policy about missed appointments and cancellations are all issues related to the *therapeutic frame*. Some therapists are uncomfortable about enforcing their policies about these issues for fear of upsetting their patients. However, addressing them can be key in dealing with subtle defenses that can undermine therapy.

Tony regularly keeps his appointments, although on a few occasions throughout therapy when we have rescheduled the time he has forgotten. He has been in therapy now for about five years. Initially, it was common for him to be five to 10 minutes late for his appointment. I explored this with Tony and suggested that he might feel uncomfortable getting here early and waiting for me in the waiting room.

Therapist: It seems you have this habit of arriving at least a few minutes late to therapy consistently.

Tony: It's not just here. It's everywhere in my life. I rush from one thing to the next and think I will have more time than I actually do.

Therapist: You describe it as though you have no control over it.

Tony: I don't, really. It's always been like this for me.

Therapist: I don't think it's beyond your control, actually. It sounds like something that has become habitual in your life, and habits can be hard to break. You're obviously very bright, and I'm sure you're capable of estimating the time different activities take in your life and how long travel will take. I wonder if there's more to it. I wonder if getting here early and having time to reflect on what you want to discuss in therapy might be uncomfortable for you?

Tony: So you're saying I wouldn't like getting here early? That it would be uncomfortable? I don't think so.

Therapist: Perhaps. Any thoughts?

Tony: I'd love to get places early . . . I think.

Therapist: But you don't do it.

Tony: Now that you say that . . . the idea of sitting in the waiting room waiting for our appointment to begin feels a little . . . desperate or something.

Therapist: Desperate?

Tony: Like that guy who needs his therapist so bad he gets there early. Maybe that guy in the movie *What about Bob?*[6] who follows his therapist around.

---

6. A 1991 comedy film about an irritating patient (played by Bill Murray) who follows his psychiatrist (played by Richard Dreyfuss) on vacation.

Therapist: So maybe getting here early would be a statement that therapy is important to you, and it feels a bit needy or desperate to value therapy like that.

Tony: Exactly! It seems a little pathetic.

Therapist: It's interesting how you have made being conscientious about being here on time an indication of pathetic neediness.

Tony: Well, when you say it like that it seems ridiculous . . . [There is a fairly long pause here, about 1 or 2 minutes but feels much longer.] I think there is something empowering about people waiting for me. When I get to surgery, I am usually the last one scrubbed in. When I come into the OR they are all waiting for me. It's like the important guy has arrived. I've sensed that before. In fact, I remember being conscious of that even as an intern. When the resident comes in to the OR it's Go time. Nothing happens without him.

Therapist: So if you were to get here early that would all be reversed. You would be waiting for me. I become THE MAN, and you are less than that . . . just waiting for someone more important.

Tony: Yeah, that's it. That feels pretty shitty when you say it. I remember as a kid waiting for the doctor in the waiting room. It seemed like forever. Who knew that one day I'd be that guy they are waiting for. I became that guy.

Therapist: Yes, the waiting doesn't feel good at all to you, so you give away time that you pay for to feel good. But you are actually cheating yourself of the opportunity to slow down a moment to consider how you are feeling before we start, which would make the session more productive.

Tony: So you don't think I'm using the sessions productively?

Therapist: It sounds like you easily heard that as a criticism.

Tony: Well, this is interesting, but I don't think it's going to change my habit of being late. It sounds like it might irritate you.

Therapist: Good move. [I laugh.] I notice how you shifted the focus to me there. You know, there may be a time or two when I feel some irritation but to be honest, you are giving me free time when you come late. It gives me those five extra minutes. I can always use a few extra minutes. [I smile . . . he smiles also.]

Tony: We'll see.

Over the next few weeks he still arrives a few minutes late. I begin the session accordingly.

Therapist: I see you are concerned about my schedule and are generously giving me a few extra minutes for myself. That's very kind of you but you really don't have to look out for me that way. [I'm teasing him . . . and he knows it and seems to like it. He often teases me when he thinks I'm getting too serious.]

Tony: Glad I could be of help.

In the following weeks Tony starts arriving on time and yes, even a few minutes early. It is now rare for him to be late for a session. Over the first few years of treatment, there has been a lot of sexual acting out, and Tony has been having a great deal of difficulty managing his life. Problems with his wife and at work have been commonplace, he has been making poor financial decisions, and he has avoided paying his taxes for three years.

Unconscious Process

For a client with narcissistic tendencies, the idea of an unconscious can feel very threatening. It causes him to feel vulnerable, believing that his mind could reveal something personal about which he is unaware. So when interpretations are made to shed light on an unconscious process, the effort is usually dismissed initially. Sometimes it is only revisited in a later session with a self-attribution as if the patient has had that notion all along. Self-attribution preserves a sense of safety and control. Here again, the unconscious is working to protect the patient from unauthorized access to his mind, even though that access is illusory. It is best to time interpretations when they address something on the edge of consciousness (in the pre-conscious). The therapist's timing and sensitivity are important.

The other way to witness the unconscious process in action is observing a patient who focuses exclusively on one symptom to avoid another around which there is greater shame.

Tony often recites the frequency of his masturbation or his usage of pornography. However, he seems to be in complete denial about his other acting out behaviors, which are generally much more destructive. He says that he feels good if he goes the whole week without masturbating but in the next breath casually mentions that his bank account is overdrawn and that he hasn't filed an income tax return for three years. He may take pride in the fact that he hasn't had an orgasm while masturbating for 30 days but downplays homosexual encounters in which he has received oral sex. He feels he is being faithful and honoring his marriage vows to his wife because he is more attracted to women than men. When I gently question whether his wife might feel differently about the matter, he dismisses me as if he never heard me. When I bring his attention to his dismissal, he gets angry. This tells me that I have been pushing too hard and so I step back and resume interpreting his vulnerability.

Empathy and Empathic Failures

Generally, with a patient who has narcissistic defenses, it is best to go the extra mile to make sure to speak from an empathic state of mind. These clients have very sensitive antennae when it comes to detecting a lack of empathy toward them. If there is any hint of criticism in vocal tone, the patient may seem to be compliant, but they may not have taken in the words and may have stiffened into a more protected state of mind and body. Many narcissistic patients have received little empathy or attunement from their parents. Once a therapist has established sufficient rapport with a patient, some teasing may be appropriate, as long as it is among the mutually accepted terms of engagement. Although some would argue that it is defensive (and at times we would agree), such a form of communication is often used with his friends and colleagues and may allow the patient to hear things that might normally make him bristle. It's like a teaspoon of sugar to help make the medicine go down more easily.

For the therapist, this is a matter of intuition and developing a certain feel for timing and subtle shifts in the relational dynamic. If the patient with narcissistic vulnerabilities feels that you are laughing at him, he can feel humiliated and strike back with anger or withdraw. Sometimes an attempt to make an interpretation makes it clear how open the patient will be. He may dismiss you simply by saying something like, "No, that's not it," and then continue as if you've said nothing. It's important to know when to let it go and when to pursue it. If you think he's not ready for what you have to say, either let it go or point it out. Here's an example of the latter approach.

Therapist: Did you notice that? I think you dismissed me without even hearing what I said.

Tony: No, I didn't notice that. What did you say?

Therapist: You really didn't hear me?

Tony: No I didn't. I think I was making a point. You kind of interrupted me.

Therapist: Perhaps I did interrupt you. I think part of your mind heard me. I said [insert brilliant comment here] and you told me I was wrong. I think part of you was uncomfortable about what I was saying to you, so you moved along quickly to soothe yourself by putting it in the past so as not be disturbed by it.

Tony: Well, if I did it, then my mind is more clever than I thought.

Therapist: Yes, I think it is.

Tony: Well, here is what I think about what you said . . .

Countertransference Reactions[7]

Tony had been in treatment for about two years when he elaborated about the moment he confessed to his wife about his sexual escapades with other men. He and his wife were having sex and he was at the height of his sexual pleasure, on the verge of climax, when he blurted out, "I want you and Mark to suck my dick." She was puzzled at first. Mark was a friend of theirs who was at their home for dinner that evening. When she asked him about it, he admitted to her that he likes the idea of having men suck his cock. At first she didn't seem to believe him, but he insisted that it was true and revealed some details of acting out with a man the week prior. She was understandably horrified when she started to realize that he was telling the truth, pushed him off of her, and jumped up out of the bed. She looked at him for a moment then began to yell at him. Surprisingly, this aroused him and he began to masturbate while she was calling him a "faggot" and a "disgusting queer." Somehow, he continued to find this arousing and masturbated to orgasm while she was doing her best to devalue and shame him.

---

7. We use the term *countertransference* to refer to the emotional, physical, behavioral, and cognitive responses of the therapist to the patient. They hinder treatment if not analyzed, but if explored they can open up the treatment and provide valuable insights about the mind of the patient.

Shame, or the feeling of being very naughty, had achieved an erotic value all its own in some type of complicated reaction formation (Freud, 1894). According to psychoanalytic theory, *reaction formation* is a defense mechanism in which unacceptable or threatening thoughts, feelings, or behaviors are denied and replaced with their opposite.

> My countertransference is triggered. I find myself thinking, "Who gets aroused by being yelled at and shamed?" I feel as though I will never be able to relate to this man. How will I help him if I don't understand what is happening in his mind at these moments? I feel as though I am sitting with an alien from another universe. His mind has developed a bizarre way to transform the negative affect of shame into something that is desired and further excites him. As he later develops a therapeutic alliance with me and begins to feel safe, he reveals some other manifestations of this dynamic. Once, in college, his roommate walked in on him masturbating and it turned him on.
>
> I struggle to understand him and then I remember an experience from my own life when I was a teenager. One day at football practice, a fellow player, who I shall call Bill, was talking to a group of us about when he went to the house of our second-string linebacker, Randy. After Randy's mother told him he was upstairs in his room, Bill went up. He opened Randy's bedroom door and found him masturbating in his room. I'm sure both were horrified, but somehow, as we were listening to the story, another player suggested a clever nickname for Randy. "From now on, we should call him 'Jerk,'" he suggested, as in 'jerking off.' We all laughed but I remember being horrified. The nickname stuck, and for the rest of our high school years he was known as Jerk. I empathized with Jerk, the boy formerly known as Randy. I think, what if that had been me? Randy became known as "Jerk" to those of us who were supposed to be his friends. He did nothing more than the other 95% of us were doing, but he got caught.
>
> In the session with Tony, I am engaged in a reverie, trying to imagine it was me that was caught by my friend masturbating in my room at home. I imagine my teenage self being flooded and overwhelmed with shame. I feel desperate to find relief from this soul-crushing terror. After our session, on the

> drive home from the office, my creative mind finds a solution. I try to imagine that a beautiful woman is turned on by the thought of me masturbating. It doesn't come naturally for me. I picture her coming in through the door and discovering me in my room. There is an awkward moment, but then she starts to get aroused. I don't stop, I continue masturbating and eventually after watching for a few minutes she starts to take her clothes off and masturbates beside me, adoring my penis. That's it! I now have a possible glimpse into how Tony could transform the shame of being caught masturbating, or cheating on his wife, into an erotic experience.
>
> This allows me to begin to imagine a scenario in which it could be arousing for Tony to be in this situation with his wife. She is trying to shame him and is venting her hurt and disappointment and anger at him in the worst possible way, but Tony has found a way to turn around shame and its impact in his mind. She is yelling at him, but not because she is disgusted with him. He imagines that she is actually aroused at the thought of him receiving oral sex from a man. It is her sexual passion that causes her to yell. She can barely contain the pleasure she feels in her body. He has always wanted this from her. Her lack of sexual interest in him is so painful, but now he has found a solution. He must disregard the reality of his wife at that moment and imagine her as a "bitch in heat." The more he masturbates, the angrier and more aroused she becomes and the harder he becomes. Of course, this is why the relationship ultimately failed: It was based on fantasy, not reality. Tony didn't see her clearly and dramatically underestimated her negative reaction to the revelation of his cheating with other men. She didn't feel he understood her and felt unsafe with him, because when he disregarded her reality it actually did make him unsafe for her.

What is the point of all this? We believe that one of the constant struggles in our work is to find some small potential for empathy within ourselves when our patients describe behaviors to us that we may think disgusting. Sometimes interventions fall flat with our patients. Technically we may say the right words, but they slip off our patient like water off a duck's back. In trying to unpack the situation, we often realize that our state of mind was not empathic. We were not speaking to the patient with understanding. We were delivering a technically correct intervention from a detached, analytic, and nonemotional position, perhaps even an elevated or superior one. The most powerful and effective words we can speak to our patients come from an open, attuned state of mind. A therapist must strive to speak in the session only after attaining that state of mind. Sometimes it takes some mental contortions, as in the example cited earlier. It often takes a great deal of patience on the part of the therapist.

A great illustration of patience of this sort is a scene in the movie *The Horse Whisperer*.[8] Robert Redford, the horse trainer, stands in the field for hours waiting for the horse to approach. Sometimes we sit in our office literally for hours, waiting for our empathy to arrive and for the patient's real self to emerge.

While trying to be patient, at the same time we must consider the self-destructive aspects of the patient's behavior. Therapists must hold in their minds two conflicting points of view at the same time or do the opposite of splitting.[9] Take Tony: He finds his wife's disgust arousing, which is out of touch with reality and destructive to his marriage. This balancing act requires a lot of a therapist. We don't necessarily want to attune to the pathology but to the impaired real self that lies beneath the pathology (Roberts, 2007).

> Another challenge with Tony is to manage my reaction to his financial irresponsibility. He drives an older model Ferrari, and it seems that it is always breaking down. It's so unreliable that I find myself wanting to recommend a Honda or Toyota. He often speaks about his assets by quoting the current market value of his real estate and automobile holdings. He has managed to accumulate quite a bit of equity, but he is usually cash poor and his wallet is often empty. He usually talks about the

---

8. *The Horse Whisperer* is a 1998 film directed by and starring Robert Redford (1998), based on the 1995 novel *The Horse Whisperer* by Nicholas Evans. Redford plays the title role, a talented and intuitive trainer with a remarkable gift for understanding horses, who is working to help an injured teenager and her horse following a traumatizing accident.

9. *Splitting* is a primitive defense mechanism in which a person simplifies the self and object representations by splitting (separating) them into their good or bad components. They have difficulty perceiving themselves or others as containing both elements, so they become all good or all bad.

value of his assets when he is feeling challenged or insecure in some area of his life, such as being close to an income tax filing deadline or a property tax due date. He is in extreme credit card debt, and many of his cards are maxed out. I feel anxious as he describes being late paying his property taxes or income taxes. I feel myself wanting to help him avoid incurring steep penalties by pointing out that he'll pay more in the long run by further delays and avoidance of fiscal responsibility. It's not uncommon for him to receive foreclosure notices on one or another of his properties. He always manages to pay the bills, often only moments before his property is auctioned off on the courthouse steps. Like a magician, he pulls the rabbit out of the hat at the last moment. In consequence, he pays what seem to be huge amounts on late fees. I could never live my life this way and I feel very critical of, and anxious about, his fiscal nonchalance.

A process of *projective identification* (PI)[10] occurs when he comes in proclaiming the drastic situation with his finances. I get anxious, but he seems calm and relaxed. I contain it until I feel I can contain it no longer. As I speak up, curious about how he manages to tolerate this stress, he tells me that it's OK because he just finished an extra-long shift on call and will get a large check to cover it by the end of the week. I have been sweating for 20 minutes during our session, only to learn that he has a solution in sight. So he projects fear and anxiety, and I experience it and resonate with it. I identify with his predicament, only to learn that he has an ace up his sleeve. I feel played. Now I find myself checking out when he talks about a financial crisis brewing. There is something ego-syntonic for him about being on the edge of bankruptcy. It is as if he is proclaiming that the normal rules of adult life do not apply to him. Just like he didn't need to show up to

---

10. PI is a defense mechanism in which the person denies painful thoughts and affects and manages to induce them in the other. It may represent an attempt to externalize the problem so it feels more manageable. An entire chapter could be devoted to this subject, as psychoanalytic authors tend to use the term in many different ways. In Masterson's model, the patient denies and projects onto the therapist, who then identifies with the projection because it resonates with some elements of the therapist's internal structure. If it doesn't resonate, it's just *projection*.

> therapy on time, he doesn't have to pay his bills on time. That is for the weak ones (which in this example includes me). He likes the adrenaline of living on the edge.
>
> Another countertransference moment for me occurs when Tony describes being late for surgery. At times he acts out in the morning with a man he met online, causing him to be late for work. This generally happens when his wife is out of town and the children are at school. I find myself getting more and more anxious as he tells me about meetings with the chief of surgery at the hospital, who has been threatening to fire him if he doesn't get his act together. On one occasion when he was acting out while on call, a patient could easily have had complications, because it caused an emergency surgery to be delayed. As he describes this calmly, I feel my anger building. I wonder if I have a duty to warn officials in this situation. I later consult with an attorney, who tells me that, in this case, there is no duty to warn.

It would horrify Tony to think of his coworkers ever finding out about the numerous ways in which he acts out. He has somehow transformed this anxiety by reversing it. In private, he engages in the most disgusting and shameful sexual acts I can imagine. He once described defecating and smearing his feces all over his body while masturbating. The more he imagined the attitude of disgust or contempt of others (his wife, his coworkers, and even me), the more erotic the experience was for him. He started to carry a selfie of himself smeared in feces on his phone. He would peek at it in the hospital but apparently no one ever noticed. I think the idea of being caught excited him.

Early Attachment Issues

> In moments when I was able to attain an empathic state of mind, I began to imagine that Tony was finding eroticism in my empathy and care. Maybe he was hungry for this in a way that made him too vulnerable to express. His mother was very cold to him in childhood, and I imagined him like Harlow's Rhesus monkeys.

In the lab, Harlow's (1966) baby primates had only two model mothers made of wire mesh. One was covered with wool cloth and the other was covered with bare wire. All of them showed their preference for the cloth monkey by clinging to it. They would visit the bare wire mother only if she was the only source of food. Eventually Harlow removed the model mothers, depriving the monkeys of any socialization at all. They were given food and water only. "One of six monkeys isolated for 3 months refused to eat after release and died 5 days later. The autopsy report attributed death to emotional anorexia" (Harlow, 1966, p. 92).

> I find myself thinking about Tony as an infant in his crib after soiling his diaper. I imagine his mother preoccupied with her career and being inattentive to his need for a clean diaper. I imagine him as he gets older, tearing off his diaper in anger and smearing the feces all over the house. Of course, infants have not achieved explicit autobiographical memory, so he wouldn't know this at a conscious level, but perhaps he knows it implicitly. These reveries make it easier for me to be present with Tony as he describes his acting out. Of course, he might be tantalized by a caring other. I don't believe that Tony ever had anyone take an interest in his experience and attune to his feelings until he entered treatment for sex addiction. Sometimes this thought of Tony receiving an erotic hit from my care and concern made me feel quite uncomfortable and used by him. What if I was his emotional prostitute? He paid me and I managed to feel empathy for him. Did this turn him on? He gave some hints that this might play in our relationship.

Tony: I have to be careful in my group because sometimes I talk about my acting out and it triggers some of the other guys. And when they give too much detail about the ways they act out I find myself being triggered. Actually, I have to watch myself because sometimes I get aroused telling my own story. I think I would be kicked out of the group if anyone knew that.

Therapist: I wonder if that ever happens here?

Tony: What do you mean? That I have to be careful about what I say because it might turn you on? [He gives a wry smile and has a smirk on his face as he looks me in the eye. I think he know exactly what I am asking, but I suspect he's playing dumb.]

Therapist: [I'm not taking the bait, but I suppose I could have wondered aloud if he was playing with me and if he actually understood what I was asking.] No, I actually meant the opposite. I wonder if, when you tell me stories about acting out, it sometimes triggers you sexually?

Tony: So, you're asking if I get turned on talking to you. Gee whiz, I realize some people may find you handsome, but you're not my type. [Feeling exposed by my question, he devalues me to put the focus back on me.]

Therapist: Interesting what you did there.

Tony: I don't know what you're talking about.

Therapist: I was asking you something very intimate about yourself and you managed to change the subject to whether or not I am handsome. I suspect you did that to protect yourself. Perhaps there was something I said that cut too close to the bone that made you feel uncomfortable.

Tony: Well, I guess you are the shrink and you know how all of this works but I have to tell you I'm not turned on by you.

[I feel a bit of shame. I start to question myself, wondering if I am barking up the wrong tree. I want to respond in some clever sarcastic way, but I manage to hold on to myself and stay still, resisting the strong urge to put him in his place like he just did me.]

Masterson (2013) called this desire for revenge the talionic impulse. He would often say, "You can get better or you can get even. You can't do both." What narcissists like Tony fear most is exposure and being seen. They hide and protect the impaired real self at all costs.

[I decide it's best to say nothing at this point and eventually the conversation shifts to another subject. I floated a trial balloon to see if I could get a purchase with an interpretation. This one seemed at the moment to have fallen flat, but at the next session Tony brings it up again.]

Tony: You know I've been thinking about what you said. You asked me if I'm attracted to you. [Actually I didn't ask this but it seems to be what the patient remembers of our discussion. What I actually asked him was whether he gets triggered when he tells me about his acting out. I think if I pointed this out to him it would be too abrupt at this moment. He appears to be feeling quite vulnerable.] I think I blew you off but there are moments here . . . [There is a pause here that lasts only about one minute, but feels more like a half-hour.]

Tony: [haltingly] There have been moments . . . when I've felt triggered.

Therapist: It seems like that must be hard to talk about.

Tony: It's just uncomfortable. [He seems to be staying with vulnerability.] It's not like I think there would ever be anything that would happen between us, but there is something triggering here at times. I guess we are talking in a very intimate kind of way and maybe that's kind of what is triggering. You know . . . I don't have these kinds of conversations with anyone in my life. Not with my wife and I certainly don't have these kinds of conversations with my friends . . . [another long pause] . . . My family didn't ever talk like this. It was all superficial shit. If I were to talk sincerely to my mom or dad they wouldn't know what to do. I think it would totally freak them out. . . . I think I probably wanted it. Probably won't ever happen with them . . . but one time it would be nice if we could have an honest, sincere conversation. Never heard "I love you" from my mom or dad growing up. Actually never heard it period. Even to this day. It isn't said.

Tony's sarcasm now makes sense to me. I imagine this was the way people talked in his family. It's a safe way to talk; sarcasm protects the speaker. This feels like a significant breakthrough. Tony's starting to identify an unmet need, the need for an intimate connection with another human being.

The following week it was as if this conversation never happened. Then he relayed a very personal conversation with a man from his clinical case conference that was very meaningful for him.

After Tony's wife learned of his sexual acting out with men, she left him. The divorce was costly and protracted. He learned that she was also having an affair during the last part of their marriage. After Tony settled the divorce he seemed to settle down. He started to date and take better care of his finances. He paid more attention to his children and began to be more aware of their emotional needs. He eventually met a woman who he was very interested in. He told her that he is a sex addict and, incredibly, she didn't run in the other direction. He discussed his sexual addiction history with her, and she appreciated his honesty. She confessed a period of anorexia during college and more recent episodes of binging and purging. She agreed to get into a support group for women with eating disorders. After dating for about six months Tony invited her to move in with him. They have been living together for a few years now and have talked about eventually getting married.

On the whole, Tony is functioning much better now. Four years after he began therapy, he has largely gained control over the sexual acting out in his life. It has been 15 months since he went to a bathhouse. He hasn't acted out with men for nearly that same amount of time. Since his day is no longer focused on scheduling time to act out between surgeries, he is doing much better at work. He has a good relationship with his chief of staff and has found support in a bible study with other men at a local church. He continues to attend a weekly sex addiction recovery group as well as individual therapy. Amazingly, he is no longer in debt. The enormous amount of time in his life occupied by sexual acting out is now spent, in part, taking care of his financial affairs and paying bills. He hasn't been late on a mortgage payment for 12 months. He has cut back his therapy to once every two weeks and has discussed termination. He doesn't feel ready to quit, but there is much less acting out to report and he is generally happy with his life and his new relationship. He feels loved and cared for in a way that he never experienced before. Along with that, he has noticed a decreased need and desire for sex. Sex twice a week is now OK for him. Although he would still prefer more frequent sex, he gets more out of the relationship than just sex and feels satisfied overall.

I've also noticed a flowering of creativity in Tony's life. Lately he has been sharing with some excitement his forays into woodworking. He was able to open a half day in his schedule to take a woodworking class at the adult education school, and he is really enjoying it. His father never did anything like that around the house and conveyed to Tony that such activity was "blue collar work." Tony felt a little bit self-conscious about wanting to take the class but decided to go for it. He has brought in some of his projects, and he seems to have a natural talent. He also seems to be finding some beauty and meaning in woodworking. He spoke to me about appreciating the beauty of the wood grain as it wraps around an imperfection, finding it a good metaphor for his life and struggles.

Tony: I love the wood smell and the grain of different types of wood. When you sand it, it releases this bouquet of scents that is indescribable. And when I put the final finish on it the transformation that takes place is so cool to witness. It's hard to believe that I could enjoy something so much. Down the road, I think I'll try a piece of furniture, maybe a dining room table.

He recently remembered an old book a friend recommended about caring for the soul (Moore, 2009). He picked it up again, and it is making much more sense than it did the first time he tried to read it. He feels that it has encouraged him to look at his life with new eyes and to pay attention to things that really excite him and turn him on—not in a sexual way, but in ways that are much deeper and more satisfying. He recently told his parents that he loved them. They seemed uncomfortable, but repeated it back to him. It took a while, but it has become more comfortable for him and (I think) for them as well.

Masterson (1988) believed that one of the primary indications of a successful treatment is the flowering of creativity. Often people develop a new hobby or pick up an old one near the end of a successful treatment. I think Tony is experiencing this flowering of creativity in his many areas of his life. He seems freer. His addiction seems like a distant memory. He occasionally masturbates to pornography, but he prefers a sexual relationship with his partner. He occasionally has momentary triggers about going to the steam baths when he drives by, but these feelings pass as he drives on.

CHAPTER 4

Treatment of an Impacted Partner

We're inclined to forgive people for mistakes they make unknowingly. And I don't mean when they "aren't aware of their actions." When people make mistakes in that way, not unknowingly, but because they "aren't aware of their actions" as a result of some emotion or state of mind that isn't natural or normal for a human being—then we're not inclined to forgive them.

—Aristotle, from *The Nicomachean Ethics*

If a movement exists to de-pathologize sex addiction (including a proscription of that term), then an even fiercer attempt has been made to de-pathologize the experience of nonacting out, impacted partners. For years, typical interventions directed at partners of sex addicts reflected what has been called a co-addict model of treatment. Based on the concept of codependency promulgated by Beattie (1978) and Melody (1989) and codified into DSM terms by Cermak (1986), co-addict partners were once characterized as colluding with a sex addict's acting out behavior, rather like a spouse of an alcoholic is said to enable drinking. Examples would have included meeting the sex addict's demands for increased frequency of sex or participating in unusual sexual activity that the nonacting out partner found uncomfortable. A co-addict partner might alter her appearance to suit the addict's mercurial tastes and feel inadequate if she did not measure up in his demands for novelty. She'd note his irritability when denied sex, be in denial of his suspicious behaviors, and accept false responsibility for his mood swings. Having worked with numerous spouses of sex addicts over the years, painful denial-breaking and intervention-inducing stories like the following come to mind:

> A woman learns during a medical check-up that she has a sexually transmitted disease (STD). A nurse practitioner asks if she has had multiple partners. Nonplussed, the woman says no. Then the nurse asks the same about her husband. The woman recalls the look on that nurse's face as she asked her clinical questions: a sympathetic, piteous expression that said, "Oh you poor thing, you don't know, do you?"

"You didn't get here overnight." That pithy statement reflects a warmly intended lesson directed at co-addicts by Claudia Black (2009), a noted author on the subject of partners of sex addicts. Referring to a suffering nonacting out partner, she wrote, "Her childhood was her training ground before she entered any of her three addictive relationships. Dysfunction ruled her original family" (Black, 2009, p. 85). Exemplifying the co-addict pattern, this woman had learned the following in her upbringing: overlooking behaviors that hurt her deeply; appearing cheerful when unhappy; minimizing conflict to avoid anger; taking care of others; and not asking for help. Reading this list of habits, you might think that Black (2009) and Tripodi (2006) are describing entire generations of women, not just partners of sex addicts. After all, the listed traits recall the "hysterical" women of the 1950s and 1960s—the women that Betty Friedan (1963) addressed and defended in her feminist manifesto, *The Feminine Mystique*. In the present-day debate between therapeutic models, we hear echoes of Friedan's stand for the mostly middle-class (and white) women of her era, as well as her rebuke of classical psychoanalysis.

Co-Addict, Relational Trauma, and Psychoanalytic Models of Trauma

Over the last decade or so, what some describe as a paradigm shift has occurred; sex addiction specialists have begun referring to nonacting out partners as trauma survivors, not co-addicts

(Hentsch-Cowles & Brock, 2013; Katehakis, 2016; Minwalla, 2012; Steffens & Means, 2009; Steffens & Rennie, 2006). According to observers, the formerly accepted term assigned inappropriate responsibility to partners of sex addicts. It was based thoughtlessly on the model of alcohol codependence, implying a pattern of enabling behaviors, if not a deeper internal pathology. Some argue that partners of sex addicts do nothing akin to flushing alcohol or drugs down toilets to prevent use or "cover up" negative behaviors by making excuses on behalf of the addict to friends, family members, or employers. Although patients don't necessarily exhibit full criteria, specialists contend that impacted partners show signs of PTSD. Dissatisfied impacted partners often leave therapy plaintive about their experience being cast in pathological terms and offended that a therapist was perceiving something wrong with *them*. Trauma specialists sympathize with this frequently reported offense and alter the perspective on impacted partners. They recast the discovery of acting out as a new, shocking event, not confirmation of something passively observed but long-denied. With their own view of what happens in therapists' offices, these specialists assert that women are blamed for their partners' sex addiction. They employ tools like the Trauma Inventory for Partners of Sex Addicts (TIPSA)[1] devised by Skinner (2015) and characterize trauma as a latent construct (not directly observable). However, problems lie with qualitative, dichotomous distinctions: those who meet the criteria (via the DSM) are said to have PTSD, while those who do not meet the criteria also have the disorder (Stokes et al., 2020).

In addition to rejecting assumptions of co-addict behavior, purveyors of the trauma-based perspective, sometimes called a relational trauma (RT) model (not to be confused with relational psychoanalysis), oppose the supposition that partners are predisposed to select sex addicts as their partners. RT advocates might not attribute these suppositions to any particular source. Minwalla

---

1. Stokes et al. (2020) critique the TIPSA, observing that questionnaires contain technically problematic and empirically disordered response items, utilize vague wording, and have results that are not generalizable because only 6% of the roughly 3,000 respondents in a national administration of the questionnaire were male.

(2012) does, suggesting that they emanate from patriarchal models[2] within mental health establishments. For example, OR theory posits phenomena derived from Freud's (1914b) repetition compulsion theory to explain why co-addicts may choose partners who re-enact early childhood abuse and neglect. Actually, psychoanalysis is responsible for several ideas borrowed by sex addiction specialists. Trauma reenactment, a term that is often bandied about by therapists within sex addiction treatment, is derivative of Freud's repetition compulsion and melancholia theories, while the term induced trauma seems derivative of PI, affirmed by many as an important concept in contemporary psychotherapy (Bion, 1962; Klein, 1946; Mitrani, 2001; Schore, 1994, 2002). Sandor Ferenczi (1930, 1933), the first prominent psychoanalyst to resurrect Freud's seduction theory, affirmed the "reality" of patients' sexual traumas. He exercised a principle of indulgence, such as not insisting that patients lie on a couch so they might relax and share the memories that haunt them. Analytic terms like denial, sublimation, displacement, reaction formation, and repression are all relevant to the treatment of both sex addiction and trauma. Dissociation, a term originally coined by Janet (1889) before the advancement of psychoanalysis, is a phenomenon of consciousness concerning the bodily experience. The similar analytic concept of splitting, which pertains to ego and internal objects, is more readily expressed in words.

Psychoanalysis is primarily concerned with the study of individuals. However, OR theory, which falls under its umbrella, bears the closest resemblance to family systems theory because it contextualizes individuals, which is crucial to patient care according to system theory pioneers like Minuchin (1974). The difference is that OR

---

2. Psychoanalysis was originally a trauma-based treatment model. In his original seduction theory, Freud believed that hysterical neurosis symptoms resulted from a prior event in which an adult close to a patient had actually violated a child sexually. Initially, this wouldn't produce problems because a child is not mature enough to be aroused or troubled, but later, the defense of repression, activated by secondary sexuality, would result in symptoms. Freud famously abandoned his seduction theory in 1897, purportedly because he could not believe that perverse acts against children were as widespread as they seemed. He later advanced the theories of infantile sexuality and the Oedipal complex, believing that children indeed have sensations and thoughts that are sexual in nature and further have difficulty distinguishing fantasy from reality (Gay, 1988).

theory promotes attention to an internalized system, not to a repertoire of external techniques aimed at shaping "boundaries" between individuals. That said, our minimalist position on collateral communications (which involves less inclusion of impacted others as consultants to an individual therapy) isn't necessarily representative of psychoanalytic models. Historically, numerous psychiatrists trained in psychoanalysis have applied systemic thinking and interventions to the understanding of family conflict (Boszormenyi-Nagy, 1967, 1972; Bowen, 1966; Bowlby, 1949; Dicks, 1967). Addressing family ethics and interlocking needs, Boszormenyi-Nagy (1967, 1972) asserted that symptoms develop when trustworthiness in a family system breaks down. Bowlby (1949) described conjoint family interviews as an adjunct to individual psychotherapy and often met with impacted others in an effort to resolve treatment impasses. Lastly, and most notably, Ackerman (1966) wrote of gathering all members of a family, to encourage spontaneous self-disclosures to confront family resistance and ease the release of family secrets from behind defensive facades. We are mindful of these variant strategies, but in the context of sex addiction treatment, we think that gatherings and hearings, especially at the outset of treatment, thwart honesty more often than not. In addition, we believe that some specialist interventions are too loaded with secondary agendas.

Terms like patriarchy, paradigm shift, and victim-blaming impute a toxic, iatrogenic power structure within treatment circles, and a target demographic may infer a call to action. Plus, this call seems to hitch on the movement against gender-based violence, a reticent but somewhat transparent shorthand for male violence directed at women. A review of the annual National Victimization Survey by the US Department of Justice, which tracks both reported and unreported crimes by and against persons over the age of 12, affirms that violent victimizations have declined 71%,[3] from 79.8 per 1,000 persons in 1993 to 23.2 in 2018 (with a small rate increase from 2015 to 2018). The survey also revealed that men experience

3. Pinker (2012) takes us much further back to declare that violence, as in sudden death at the hands of others, has dramatically declined over history, despite popular assumptions to the contrary. Estimating that modern society is over 90% less violent than it was 500 years ago, he partly attributes this change to the rise of women in society. In other words, the push-back against "toxic masculinity" began centuries ago.

higher victimization rates than women for all types of violent crime other than sexual assault, including murder. You might not think this was true if you read contemporary authors like Rebecca Solnit (2020), whose anecdotes and comments (rightly) decry violence against women but imply that men face dangers in lesser numbers and that violence toward women is more acceptable to society. This is not about numbers. Actually, it may be one of those anomalies in which pundits would have us look beyond data. Or some may observe that men are four times as likely to perpetrate violence, as if this fact is relevant to identifying those at greater risk. Data clearly suggest that race and class are the salient at-risk categories for violent victimization, not gender. Contrary to what field-levelers imply, violence against women likely elicits special attention because it's more offensive to people across the sociopolitical spectrum and because sexual violence is particularly humiliating.

Narratives bleed into sex addiction treatment, so relational trauma specialists posit the word trauma as a clinical substitute for the word injustice, with some conflating sex addiction with gender violence (and possibly racial hatred) as the norm, not an exception. For example, according to one treatment website (togetherwecan heal.com), "deceptive sexuality is a form of domestic violence" that carries spiritual consequences, "shattering a person's relationships with divine systems." Really? In addition, the website specifies that Hispanic women serve as triggers of hypervigilance for nonacting out partners. The proposed theory of induced trauma (Minwalla, 2012) creates a syllogistic link between trauma syndromes and sex addiction assessment. This begs the following questions: if an acting out partner does not meet the criteria, should the nonacting out partner still be assigned the label sex addiction–induced trauma? Might the term sex addiction–induced trauma be used regardless of what label is assigned the acting out person? Could we then have infidelity-induced trauma, or alcoholism-induced trauma, or gambling-induced trauma? We observe that addictive patterns not directly relating to sex do not elicit the same levels of intense reaction or diagnosis-approximating clusters of PTSD symptoms. Fortunately, for an unfolding treatment, such terms might not even matter.

Actually, terms do matter, because language both validates and weaponizes, with some in our field making claims that might have caused Joseph McCarthy to blush. Proponents of the Relational Trauma model bristle at the sex addict claim of victimless behavior, seeking to recast roles and divide interventions. Perpetrator and victim appear as Manichean designations that mark divides, simplifying treatment. For some practitioners, porn use is tantamount to rape, which is akin to the vegan contention that meat eating is murder. Grounded clinicians craft their rhetoric with care whether they support these positions or not. In collegial exchanges, we hear them paraphrase their denunciations of narcissism, patriarchy, or the "toxic masculinity" of the core sex addict population. With male patients, they speak from the other side of their mouths, employing "man-to-man" confrontations, patronizing supposedly core masculine principles like responsibility to family or personal integrity. The addict has victimized his loved one or failed in his manly commitments. On the one hand, this might seem a worthwhile stab at cognitive dissonance, an effort to expose the disparity between acting out behavior and the purported values of the patient. But the tactic is not just emasculating. It is also disingenuous because it pretends an affinity for violated principles that many clinicians deem old-fashioned and false. A strategy of defense penetration is indicated largely because of an apparent or presumed collapse in values. At the same time, nonacting out partners receive a trauma survivor's prescription, which contra-indicates confrontation because the survivor's "defenses," including splitting, are considered necessary for self-care.

The clinical protest aimed at sex addiction advocates for victims. However, despite the prevalence of intersectional rhetoric, the focus in treatment ultimately lands on the impacted partner more than the plights of objectified women in porn or economically marginalized prostitutes. Therefore, the average provider takes a foot off the pedal of social justice. Still, the narrowed context is painful enough for the would-be sex addict: while enacting a role that is in one respect ego-syntonic (better to be a perpetrator than a victim), acting out partners generally accept that they have betrayed monogamous agreements and have caused a distress-inducing breakdown of trust via their lies and denials. Across secular therapeutic models, secrecy and lies are the principal sins of human behavior. The result is a partner who is disoriented by insecure narratives and lost about what is true. It's no wonder that (typically) she is disorganized in her accusations, her suspicions, and her talionic, helicoptering scrutiny of her male partner. It's not clear whether RT adherents encourage this latter behavior more than their disparaged co-addict model colleagues. We've read numerous RT blogs that refer to the profile of nonacting out partner behaviors as "normal," while others appear to espouse the co-addict model and use the word "natural" to describe the same profile. The former term implies socialization, while the latter suggests something that comes from nature, but the essential message is the same.

Some RT specialists appear to echo the now maligned co-addict perspective, not to mention psychoanalytic theory. A prominent example of partner witness literature is the Steffens and Means (2009) book, *Your Sexually Addicted Spouse*. Here, discovery of sex addiction (based on spousal assessments, not those of professionals) is a traumatic event, but partners also suffer from complex trauma derived from attachment injuries that have become ingrained in personality, according to the authors. Their case examples refer exclusively to women who felt ignored as children and were raised to take care of others, priming themselves for lives of self-denial, or "people-pleasing." This seems to say the same thing that proponents of the co-addict model are saying: experienced trauma is influenced both by the nature of an event and by previous exposure to other (perhaps unrelated) traumatic events (Follette et al., 1996). Steffens and Means (2009) suggest that many sex addict partners' traumas, while reactivated by the sexual acting out and lies of a partner, contain an excess of affect with an etiology that predates the discovered sexual betrayal. This would appear to assign some responsibility to impacted partners. We do not mean responsibility for the partner's sexual acting out, but for understanding their own undefined yet discernible role in a longer-standing problem. This undefined role is not characterized as codependency, much less a personality disorder, though some characterizations seem to draw fine lines between the two. Indeed, the term complex trauma appears to merge the concepts of trauma and personality disorder while emphasizing the more palatable term trauma, likely because it connotes victimization rather than pathology.

Trauma Profile and the Reconfigured Environment: Labels, Boundary Agreements, and "Full Disclosure"

The assignment of trauma resonates with partners who feel that they have been deceived repeatedly and betrayed in intimacy (as in cheated on). However, not all partners equate porn use with infidelity. Indeed, partners of sex addicts do not react uniformly to any of the misbehaviors discussed here. Many are distraught or angry in response to affairs or prostitute-seeking, while others seem either resigned or moderately sympathetic about their partner's "addiction." Some even seem nonchalant. Yet each of these responses can be seen as a defense. According to Van der Kolk, McFarlane, and Weisath (1996), while trauma generally results from an external event of certain intensity, an individual's response determines whether or not an event is actually traumatizing. In this way, the question, "What is traumatic?" parallels the question, "Is sex addictive?" As stated earlier, it's not so much the *agent provocateur* (as Freud put it, the drug, the behavior, or the event) as the internal and behavioral responses that determine the affliction. This seems to generate confusion among patients, with some seeking help, wondering if sex is intrinsically addictive, or if sex addiction "naturally" induces trauma syndromes, while taking only a glancing look within to find the real answers. What would lead a person to accept the idea of an internal, context-crossing problem, whether they are an acting out partner or a nonacting out partner?

Those who do not think this is the charter of treatment are more likely drawn to practitioners who will cast them as victims. Better yet, they seek out those who characterize them as survivors, a term that suggests aspirational qualities, empowerment, and hope. The survivor characterization is ego-syntonic (harmonious with their goals and self-image) but retains the "victim" connotation that externalizes blame. Another purpose of this much sought-after approach is a desire for structure and education; defining terms clears the air of noisome, fault-diffusing ambiguity. Homework will be given. A recovery plan will be devised, based on collaboration. This strategy, if carried out well, will soothe anxiety. It will also contain the flooding responses of the traumatized by recognizing that dissociation, a primitive capacity for shutting down emotion, is purposeful if not intentional. A crudely executed treatment strategy might offhandedly excuse defensive reactions to trauma, even though PTSD criteria suggest that afflicted individuals' responses are distorted. One example pertains to the symptom of hyperarousal. If triggered to anger, an impacted partner may cite her trauma to justify verbal abuse, or she may mirror the addict by not talking or even thinking about problems relating to sex. She may expel a partner from the bedroom or the home for sexual misdeeds or tertiary sins, behaviors that may seem innocuous to the average observer.

Like a soldier with PTSD, the betrayed partner extends her trauma beyond the appropriate context—beyond the war zone, so to speak. Anything that is thinly reminiscent of past events can stir panic and hostility, making aggressive responses seem necessary. RT therapists may support these responses, raising the anti-gaslighting alert that privileges these fearful actions. They may advise sex addicts to move out of their homes, at least temporarily, even when violence is not a risk factor. While the pretext for such recommendations is always the trauma of the betrayed partner or the subtler belief that traumatized persons—like addicts—suffer from an ever-relapse-able syndrome, it's hard to believe that moral outrage isn't a truer source of such "boundary setting" directives. A philandering husband has broken his vows and has thus forfeited property rights. He merits unhinged diatribes from a partner who needs to discharge her oft-choked feelings, with vitriol if not violence, for as long as they are cathartic. Ferenczi (1930) dubbed such eruptions of emotion paleocatharsis, a temporary facsimile of release, to distinguish them from a truly cathartic ending. Those who claim that religious or "family" values interfere with sex addiction treatment might take note. They may have called out bias concerning diagnosis, but they overlook how malicious actions are sanctioned by trauma-speak.

Across blog articles and self-help books that comprise a bulk of sex addiction literature, "sex-positive" critics of sex addiction treatment appear to compete with RT advocates for positions of ethical correctness. Possibly at odds, they seem allied but speak past one another, like rival factions within a generally like-minded polity. RT therapists call for therapeutic separation, a euphemism for asking the sex addict to leave his home. In their study, Corley, Pollard, Hook, and Schneider (2013) reported that close to 30% of addicts moved out of their homes or their bedrooms, compared to roughly half as many impacted partners. Based on treatment demographics, it's inferable (though not proven) that a significantly higher number of male sex addicts leave or are asked to leave their homes compared to FSLAs. Some RT therapists proclaim a "partner bill of rights" with respect to self-care or household boundaries—another euphemism. Or they might espouse the use of porn-blocking or monitoring software with names like "Covenant Eyes" or the matronly-sounding "Net Nanny." The religious, monogamous, virtue-signaling overtones of such tools are obvious and are perhaps reserved for married heterosexual couples, not for members of LGBTQ+ communities. Otherwise, it's difficult to understand why such blatantly moralistic positions are not excoriated by those in the sex addiction treatment field who lament the pathologizing of sex—not just infidelity or porn use, but also paraphilias like cross-dressing and sado-masochism. Kort (2015) and Klein (2012) criticize sex addiction specialists across media, claiming that they want to impose puritanical beliefs and eliminate behaviors that are traditionally considered deviant. But what do such critics think of RT advocates who park their judgments behind the righteous backs of the betrayed? What do sex-positive critics think or feel with respect to impacted partners? Are those partners puritans also? Or are the sex-positive dissenters reluctant to go there, wary of being tagged as "victim blamers"?

Participants in residential or short-term intensive treatments that require attendance several nights per week may be sent home with instructions for sustained abstention from acting out, along with prescriptions for improved trust between partners such as honesty or boundary agreements. There is value in spelling out agreements. Consider these examples:

- "Checking in" while one or both partners are traveling.
- Negotiating a certain degree of phone or internet monitoring by a nonacting out partner, assuming that person is agreeable to reading emails and checking junk files and search histories.
- Facilitating an agreement that attempts to contact—and attempted contacts from—former lovers be disclosed by acting out partners.

However, not all "boundary" agreements work out:

> One couple agreed that if the acting out partner (the man) would disclose instances of "slips" within 24 hours, he'd receive amnesty in the form of appreciation for honest disclosure, plus a diminution of negative consequences. He'd be exiled from the bedroom but not the house. The thinness of this pact was exposed when the man obeyed the time frame but failed to disclose some porn use prior to the couple having sex during that same period. When he disclosed

the true chronology of events the woman was irate, claiming that their intimacy (which she'd requested) was based on a false pretext and therefore constituted another lie. Context over temporality. Suffice it to say that the "yeah, buts" did not win the argument.

A dose of Realpolitik features in one staple of sex addiction treatment: the facilitated "full disclosure" activity. The term is a misnomer because the protocols for these multisessions plus behind-the-scenes therapist summits tend to prescribe factual disclosures rather than insight-oriented opinions. So, despite the diligent efforts applied, these exercises are actually constricted. Corley and Schneider (2002) provided guidelines for therapists working with sex addicts and co-addicts (the latter a commonly used term at the time of their study). The authors' observations echoed the commonplace opinion that secrets relating to infidelity should be revealed promptly if couples therapy is to proceed. However, they offered that certain factors confound this prescription in cases of sex addiction. For example, addicts are prone to staggered disclosures—they reveal acting out behaviors in increments. In addition, due to the volume and longevity of an acting out pattern, some addicts may legitimately not recall all that they have done, or they may have been in altered (e.g., intoxicated[4]) states when acting out sexually. As a result, the disclosure of acting out behaviors between addict and co-addict ought to be managed, according to these authors. They recommended that letters should be written and an acting out history outlined, including not only sexual acts but also acts of deceit or manipulation (of the impacted partner). The impacted partner should take the lead in declaring goals but may be warned against seeking information about the following areas: specific sexual activities, locations of activities, or the contact numbers or addresses of the addict's acting out partners. Lastly, the exercise climaxes with an apology by the addict for the acting out pattern.

4. This is a confusing point because it suggests a separate state of intoxication from that attributed to a sexual acting out episode. Patrick Carnes's (1991) definition of sex addiction indicates that a sexual acting out episode itself constitutes a trance-like, mood-altered, or dissociated state. If the authors agree with this definition, the indication of substance intoxication as the source of memory distortion seems redundant.

This rough outline of tasks, whether methodically prepared or not, whether heard with surprise or with foreknowledge (some information will be a shock to hear at any point), doesn't necessarily prevent meltdowns between partners, or the unfolding of posturing stratagems. In treatment, the sexually acting out person may be told he is a sex addict, and perhaps further informed that he has a personality disorder along the narcissistic or antisocial personality continuum. If the would-be addict is female, borderline personality is the more likely diagnosis. Schizoid personality, a unicorn to most sex addiction specialists we meet, will likely be ignored, or else cast as introversion, or perhaps an "on the spectrum" autistic disorder if a withdrawn pattern of behavior is observed. The impacted partner might be told she has sex addiction induced trauma, another non-DSM assessment label symbiotically tied to a sex addiction assessment, suggesting the former assessment is predicated on the latter (if addiction, then trauma). This implies that any and all dysfunction proceeds exclusively from discovery of a partner's acting out behaviors, a position at odds with analytic thinking about trauma.

Ostensibly, the dichotomous positions assigned at the outset of treatment are meant to soften and flex over time. What our field is truly saying about complex trauma is that trauma associated with discovery of sex addiction is likely a reenactment of an unconscious imprint, not simply an intrusive, aberrant life event of adulthood. This is not a "victim-blaming" assertion. Instead, it acknowledges a patient's complexity, plus historical context. We suppose it's possible that inflammatory designations of perpetrator and victim are intended as stop-gap measures to enjoin impacted partners and keep them coming back until such a time that a more nuanced, authentic story might unfold.

There are sound reasons why the reenactment pitch isn't delivered at the outset of treatment. First, as often articulated by trauma specialists, it's a matter of what impacted partners are prepared for and thus able to integrate into self-identity; this pertains to unconscious experiences not directly conveyed in words. This view echoes what Freud (Freud & Breuer, 1895) originally termed deferred action, or *apres coup* (actually a translation of the German word *Nachtraglich*). This term, a remnant of his original seduction theory, suggests that disturbing memories (which are invariably sexual in Freud's theory) are repressed until later, when the original meaning arrives too late to act upon. History becomes altered as patients think, rethink and then—often to their surprise—reremember. Until then, the symptoms (the acting out behaviors) are reenactments regarded as cathartic (if misinterpreted) or hung on to as ego-syntonic defenses. In either case, they serve as release for the patient.

Upon discovery, it's natural that non-acting out partners experience episodic trauma (shock), which affects what information they can take in emotionally. This may be quite limited when a traumatic effect is immediately felt, let alone when it is dissociated, or "deferred," as is typical in cases of childhood or chronic trauma patterns. Wanting to resolve conflict quickly ("get past it"), would-be sex addicts tend not to consider other, secondary factors. What the acting out person has known about their own behavior has generally been unknown by their significant other, so the putatively reparative discussions and disclosure exercises of early treatment do not begin on an equal footing. The impacted partner needs time plus a reconfigured environment to absorb their "new" reality, while the person with the loosening secrets needs to accept defeat of their reality-denying habit. However, that a post-discovery living environment is reconfigured via boundary agreements or disclosure exercises doesn't mean that a dominantly unilateral pattern of abuse or neglect is accepted over time.

Some cases do not merit suggestions that a problem is mutually generated, or symbiotic, but in our experience, most cases of purported sex addiction are not so facile. When feelings run high, especially outrage stemming from perceived injustice, the tendency is to sympathize with the unwitting and "get tough" with those who have transgressed traditional morality or whatever prevails as modern ethics in 2020. Furthermore, addicts are often unsympathetic. They may tell you the sky is green just to get you off their backs, and many don't have opinions about the social impact of their behaviors—just about whether they've done what you say they've done. The accusation is the thing: the persecutory fear. Therefore, it's tempting to choose sides, to decide who is right and who is wrong, and facilitate contrition when it's ripe, before shame and guilt subside and defensive entitlements resume. Contrarily, it's also easy to conclude that systemic interventions, like boundary-setting and disclosure exercises, necessarily constitute "taking sides."

Some terms draw attention to the fallacy of narrowly defined roles. For example, from the field of chemical dependency, there's the scapegoat figure. This may be an acting out person whose behaviors represent a worthy protest or someone who is oppositional, abusing drugs to break a family's code of decorum. Acting out by the scapegoat draws attention to a family problem, whether observed or hidden. Another example is the so-called identified patient (IP) figure in psychiatric care. The IP's problems simultaneously draw attention to and deflect from the problems of a disordered family. Throughout our industry, the notion that a disorder is systemic rather than strictly individualized is a popular and often-employed standard. It represents a baseline objection to fundamental attribution error, to binary thinking, or splitting.

The problem is that scapegoats and IP constructs refer tacitly to social or familial underdogs, such as adolescents. However, since the majority of acting out partners in sex addiction treatment are men and the majority of impacted partners are women, standard systems theory labels are forgotten in the face of social change initiatives. As suggested earlier, many female therapists may be wary of referring acting out female patients to "stigmatizing" sex addiction treatment, while at the same time lamenting the lack of resources for sexually addicted women. In addition, they may promote revision of contemporary mores, because they do not consider the sexually addictive behaviors of men and women to be "morally equivalent." In other words, men's actions are worse. When asked why fewer women seek sex addiction treatment, our female colleagues tend to project on this point, theorizing—without credible evidence—that impacted male partners are less "forgiving" than impacted women. More substantively, these colleagues cite reports of physical abuse suffered by sexually acting out women, which by implication contra-indicate the engagement of nonacting out male partners in supportive therapeutic efforts. Therefore, the treatment of impacted partners is primarily aimed at women, which inclines the field toward the following conclusions: female partners of sex addicts are traumatized figures whose secure attachment and trust in a deep, intimate bond has been broken. Male partners of female sex addicts are speculatively dangerous figures whose economic privilege affords them more freedom to exact revenge instead of seeking treatment for their partners. Concerns about their potential for domestic violence often supersede concerns about gaslighting, and in keeping with a familiar conception, these men are not so much traumatized as narcissistically wounded.

Alternative Profiles of Impacted Partners

We've treated more partners of sex addicts than we ever thought we would. Our surprise stems from a belief that female therapists are best positioned to treat FSLAs or female partners of sex addicts because they are women. A few chances have come our way to lead women's sex addiction partners/betrayed partners/sexual-addiction-induced trauma survivor support groups, but we've generally seen such patients in the context of individual or couples therapy—contexts in which our gender has not seemed as controversial. Perhaps this implies something about the purpose of groups framed around gender, or a clinical or social issue that is framed around gender. With respect to the group dynamic, perhaps it's not so much that women know or understand more about the perspective of their own sex, or that a corresponding truism exists within men's groups. Maybe it's that men and women have things to say that can be best said in a group format (this idea is explored further in Chapter 5). Still, seeking refuge from the opposite sex is not the purpose of therapy. We have retained numerous female clients over the years precisely because they want an opposite object experience rather than the safety, comfort, or familiarity of a presumed gender mirror.

Many impacted partners enter therapy with distorted beliefs borne of previous experiences in therapy, or their reading of self-help literature. Holden (2005) states, "men are prone to physical behavior that includes drinking, drug abuse and violence, whereas women are more likely to internalize, leading to depression and disorders such as anorexia" (p. 1574). Some women read or hear variations on such views and infer that men have tantrums, get drunk or stoned, and become destructive when stressed, and women cope with stress by getting depressed, or by protesting meekly and then retiring to their beds. It should come as no surprise that many women emerge from therapy feeling exhorted to turn the tables in their relationships. However, women who we've treated notice that something is missing from such conceptions. They feel patronized by a dominantly sympathetic narrative, wanting instead to be known more fully, warts and all. For sure, they want their betrayal or trauma acknowledged and their anger toward their male partners validated. At the same time, there's an implicit meaning in their choice of a male therapist. They want a man to show tolerance toward their anger, perhaps setting limits on expression when such tolerance has been demonstrated. They need male therapists, perhaps ones with a Kleinian ear for aggression, to observe and experience the prickly "mean girls" inside of them.

Given the freedom we feel to avoid educating patients about the latest in orthodox terminology and narratives, we can instead listen for how women describe their own experiences and explore their intended and unintended meanings. Ferenczi (1930), in paraphrasing Freud's "recommendations of technique," wrote that psychoanalysis should provide a tension between nongratification and freedom of speech. Recalling Bion (1962), whose theory of PI expanded upon Klein's (1946) conception, we see the therapist's role as analogous to a mother's early role. We must accept the projections of bad experiences, then modify them so they become tolerable. Again, we acknowledge that an impacted partner's experiences are not uniform, as there is no requisite or standard response to learning that a partner has been keeping important secrets about sex, possibly for years.

Nonetheless, we have observed some patterns. Partners that present more stoically tend to be older and have long since looked the other way with respect to porn use, and sometimes concerning the use of prostitutes. However, they tend to draw the line on affair partners, especially other women who may be known to them. These impacted partners seem less inclined to describe themselves as traumatized. Moral indignation, rather than an emotional dissembling of a formerly understood reality, seems to take center stage. Those who are rendered financially or legally vulnerable because of another's offenses, regardless of their age or propensities, tend to focus on the matters that have disrupted their world, such as managing finances or determining whether relocation from the home or community is necessary.

Younger female partners of sex addicts tend to be angrier and more humiliated, making them more frenetic with or controlling of the treatment process, including aspects of a partner's social life such as social media or bank account activity. Unlike older partners, younger women may not have at their disposal the shame-lessening rationale that sex addicts are typically drawn to younger women. A younger woman might infer a greater failure when a partner is acting out. She might consider whether she is insufficiently attractive in an intrinsic way, not changeably because of time. This is, of course, damaging to self-esteem. Younger women more commonly say things like, "I did everything I could, had sex with him whenever he wanted, did what he wanted." Declining sexual interest after the childbearing years, fatigue, or painful intercourse due to menopause may mitigate the outrage of a middle-aged or older woman toward a husband's acting out, but such pretexts are less available to younger women. Also, because younger women have a longer life ahead of them, they perhaps wish to bear more children with their partners, hearing their so-called biological clocks ticking. Short of leaving and starting again with someone else, such women face pressure to resurrect a sex life that has been broken by a chronic problem, not just an isolated incident of infidelity or a discrete phase of porn use. Therefore, treatment—with its unclear assessments and unpromising prognoses, its prescriptions like "learn skills of self-care and seek support," and its facilitation of "full" disclosures that deluge partners with ugly, previously unknown truths—can indeed be overwhelming.

A patient approach to addressing such problems is warranted. To put it simply, conceptualizing the discovery of sex addiction as trauma inclines clinicians to slow the treatment process, which is indicated in a psychodynamic model. In consultation about a discharge plan or a referral, private clinicians often learn about prior short-term programs and procedures that incorporated an impacted partner's component. These usually involve psychoeducational presentations, and also facilitation of full disclosure of the would-be addict's acting out history between partners. In individual therapy, we hear women share their thoughts about these day-long exercises and disclosures, which they describe as torturous and mind-numbing, causing them to withdraw and feel drained and disoriented. It wasn't as if they hadn't signed up for such a process. Indeed, some had demanded to know everything as soon as possible. In retrospect, however, they report not feeling ready. Something else is called for in such cases. An immersion into their experience may be girded by boundary setting or facilitations of disclosures from acting out partners, but the unfolding process is not just a perpetual validation of protest. Space must be created for reflective thought.

We give opinions to patients to stir thinking, not to stamp authority on an idea. Consider the following question from an impacted partner: "What if I had sex with him more often?" This expresses the belief that submission to a sex addict's sexual needs would deter acting out. While sex or the lack of sex should be talked about between partners (a sign of a healthy relationship, after all), we caution that sex addiction isn't primarily about the frequency of sex, or even the quality of or novelty of sexual activity. (In addition, the implication, "I'll have sex with you to stop you acting out" is not very sexy.) Having more or better sex isn't the solution to sex addiction, we might suggest. Hasty actions, like binary labels, pander to desperation, are too dissolving of dynamic possibilities, or collapse the space needed for reflective thought. This collapsed space is already characteristic of addicts, and so it is of many impacted partners. One clue that (her) trauma is developmental rather than episodic is a repeated display of psychic equivalence, a state of mind which indicates a failure to distinguish between feeling and thought. For example, if an impacted partner is reflexively triggered by a suspicious email, it may seem as if there is no room for doubt that a suspected event has occurred. This survivalist position is understandable if the impacted partner has experienced episodic trauma. But what if this pattern of reaction persists or had manifested previously and across contexts? Fonagy and Target (1996) proposed that in normal development, concrete and "pretend" modes of thought are integrated by age four to five, enabling reflective capacity; however, this capacity is often arrested in those with developmental trauma.

We observe that the hypervigilance of impacted partners arouses feelings rather than reducing or displacing them. In this way, the hyperaroused impacted partner contrasts with the obsessive acting out or addicted figure. Freud (1894) observed that obsessives fend off distress by separating it from unbearable ideas, so that distress arises in other fields. This is a feature of repression or its subordinate defenses (displacement and reaction formation): feelings are redirected onto that which generates distress, but they don't elicit nearly as much stress as the original, unbearable idea. Or, they are reversibly transformed. Recall the description in Chapter 3 of Tony, who in therapy substituted talking about masturbation for homoerotic encounters, and later experienced his wife's disgust for him as arousing. If an impacted partner directs attention to something that stirs distress, a nonacting out partner may dissociate, or "numb out" in a manner that resembles the habits of addicts, or she may amplify the distress and extrapolate *to* the unbearable, not away from it.

Regarding sex, many impacted partners are confused, because what sex addicts appear to seek—and what impacted partners often report feeling in their intimate lives with sex addicts—doesn't actually seem like sex. For example, porn teaches counterfeit sex. In analytic terms, pornography actually represses sex, substituting a contradiction. On the one hand, porn is a distortion, depicting exaggerated positions, unblemished skin, and rigorously cleansed or even bleached private parts to eliminate disgust. On the other hand, it is controversial because it *is* real. Defying the repressive conventions of media, porn doesn't distort enough. Porn is naked, so to speak; at once bathed and uncensored, but unreal.

Psychotherapy shouldn't censor, but addressing sex with an impacted partner may be harder than talking about it with a sex addict. And it may be even harder across a gender divide. Bader (2009) writes of sex as if it were the final frontier of psychotherapy: "If men are in treatment with me long enough, they will eventually allude to some problems in their sex life" (p. 107). Talking about sex in any context doesn't happen without considerable discomfort and so it requires patience and sensitivity. Sex addiction treatment would appear to slice through barriers of resistance because of crisis scenarios, but thinking doesn't flow easily, especially in the immediate aftermath of discovered behaviors. For an impacted partner, talking about sex in private contexts has seemed tantamount to promising sex, because of past or ongoing pressure to resume having sex while feeling insecure. So, why might a therapist share ideas about porn or scopic drives with impacted partners? We likely wouldn't, but impacted partners do enter therapists' offices asking questions like "Why is he like this?"

The women we have treated say that they want truth back. This is how they would prefer to reignite closeness or learn about sex addiction. "Truth before sex" would be an apt bumper sticker for a nonacting out partner's support group. Truth about the facts, at least, if not the rationales. The rationales for sexual acting out stagger and confound; they stir equal measures of incredulity and resignation because the disclosures are both shocking and not. "How could you . . ." The question stops because the answer is too big to digest. Inquiry might turn to minutiae, to bits and pieces that might eventually make sense as a whole story develops. Consider this:

> A couple is discussing the whereabouts of a man's car when he was out acting out, visiting an affair partner. (Discovery came in the form of a parking ticket that was carelessly disregarded, with a notice later sent to the home address and opened by the wife.) "Where did you park your car?" the wife demands. "Why didn't you pay the ticket?" she asks, suddenly matching his penchant for misplaced focus. Such conversations don't begin at a logical introduction but rather somewhere in the hazy middle. A betrayed figure is bewildered; she understands longing, lust and attraction, the lure of novelty, and certainly romance. But why hasn't time, place, commitment, and circumstance trumped her husband's impulses? Why does the mind collapse context, break down memory? "I am the car," the wife realizes. "The car is the symbol of our life, and if you can forget where you parked it then you forgot where you parked me."

You might think that mistrust because of lying or withholding is a mutually directed mistrust, no matter who is telling the lion's share of untruths. To withhold information or to tell lies to another conveys an implicit distrust in that other's capacity to understand or contain reactions to truthful information. "You can't handle the truth!" is a famous cinematic aphorism that speaks to this dynamic. Impacted partners may recognize and agree with this explanation but tend to give it little more than an academic nod, thinking the onus remains on the acting out partner to disclose his secrets, to "open up more." They may otherwise declare what Zitzman and Butler (2009) found in a modest study: 9 out of 14 wives reported that, after learning of their husband's pornography use, subsequent, voluntary disclosures lessened the loss of trust from the initial discovery. In a subsequent study, Corley et al. (2013) concluded that voluntary disclosure is positively related to relationship satisfaction; they found that honesty and clarity around disclosure of relapse, plus acknowledgment of a partner's pain, helped restore trustworthiness. However, the authors indicated that honest disclosures did not appear to be the norm in their study sample, which was comprised dominantly of committed couples whose relationships had lasted an average of 15 years.

Despite the seeming promise of restored trust, fully honest disclosures seem few and far between. In that same study, 25% of self-identified addicts reported that they had told their partners everything following initial discovery, while roughly 34% disclosed a great deal but withheld some information. (This suggested another 40% who were either confused or not truthful with researchers.) Most of the self-identified addicts in the study "never" or "rarely" disclosed acting out or relapse behaviors prior to discovery, which reinforces our suppositions about the factors that precipitate treatment. Again, splitting (keeping the good and the bad separate in the service of preservation—in this context an act of secrecy) is a stubborn defense. Telling the truth sounds simple when the task is narrowed, but what if it's not? Closer inspection reveals deep ambivalence about full-scale honesty. Do impacted partners really want to hear about potentially onerous sexual needs? Do they really want to hear criticisms of their physicality? Do they really want to hear about their partner's insecurities, lowering self-esteem, or body image issues? Do they really want to hear about fantasies and learn the explicit details about standards of desirability they cannot meet or no longer wish to meet? In response to such questions, many impacted partners prevaricate and express discomfort. Some counter, reasonably enough, that the most useful form of honesty is directed at oneself, not at another. However, they might intuit that disclosure of "facts" is just the beginning of a conversation they may not want to have. These partners usually concede that the truths they want to hear are emotional in nature, but not wishfully fantastic. They seek expressions of devotion and commitment and of the realities of aging and loss. Desire? Not so much, or—especially among older women—not anymore.

Some spouses remain isolated, cut off from the sisterly comfort of other impacted women because they don't want to be frightened by others' stories. Or, like those men who resist associations with other sex addicts because "most of them are much worse than me," these women distance themselves from comparisons, preferring denial or the dissociative haze of their trauma as conceptualized by others. Steffens and Rennie (2006) found that wives of sex addicts describe their husband's disclosures of sexual acting out as distressing events, leading to trauma-related symptom severity. Interestingly, these researchers also found that stress was exacerbated by preexisting factors, including years of marriage at the time of disclosure and previous exposures to traumatic events. Another feature of these women's trauma is the lack of support systems because cooperating with treatment prescriptions might alienate them from traditional support networks. That's consistent with another observation by relational trauma practitioners: impacted partners may feel inhibited from sharing their pain with family or friends who might judge them harshly for remaining committed to an acting out partner (rather than leaving him); for not "standing up" to toxic masculinity, or not heeding old warnings about the shady guy to whom they'd committed their life; for not protecting their children from bad influences; for letting down other women by colluding with the sex addiction "excuse." Such women may be wary of therapy or support groups, believing they will be advised to make decisions they don't want to make.

Some of the women we've counseled on these issues are beyond angry and beyond betrayed. They don't seem traumatized as that concept is typically employed. For these partners, the damage is beyond repair, whether they choose to leave their relationships or not. Some might choose to endure an ongoing détente, usually for the sake of children. In analyzing their profiles, we have observed not the dearth of forgiveness often imputed as a counter-judgment against angry women, or greater financial dependence on their partners, or any lack of loving intention, but rather an advanced self-righteousness that long predates discovery of acting out. Such women don't simply characterize themselves as loving mothers and wives; they think of themselves as *more* loving and nurturing than others. Their maternal, empathetic qualities are elite and they don't seem to register when others disagree. Also, they are largely dismissive of male biology. They don't seem interested in the significantly higher levels of testosterone that influence men's sex drives or place them "at risk" for externalizing behaviors (Schore, 2016). No different than men who contend that menstruation and menopause diminish women's rationality, these women act as if male biology renders men inferior in terms of social maturity and perhaps intelligence.

When asked what male partners are meant to do instead of an active sex life, these women have no answer. If they feel pressed they withdraw, not ready for *that* discussion. A clinician pushing this issue may soon receive a voicemail message expressing polite appreciation for services, indicating vaguely that "they" will be moving in a different direction. Other women who, for various reasons, have diminished sexual interest are more flexible. They may tolerate a partner's self-sufficiency, such as masturbation to fantasy to find sexual relief, while the more rigidly dismissive figures appear unable to tolerate this arrangement, instead wanting their male partners to retire sexually, as they have. For them, declining interest may be disguised by extolling the virtues of "emotional intimacy," by critiquing the "objectifying" nature of their partners' interest, or by using coded words like "penetrative" or "performative" to malign their partners' demands. They reject the notion that sex addiction reflects self-medication or dissociation; both concepts are dismissed as psychiatric sophistry, the aforementioned "excuses." They insist that sexual misbehavior is conscious in every sense: calculated, pleasure-seeking, and above all, revealing of a weak character.

The Anti-Honeymoon

Whether a couple resumes an active sex life or not, discovery of an acting out pattern is often followed by a period we call the anti-honeymoon. Sex enters a moratorium during which addiction is no longer the excuse for more sex but rather the pretext for halting sex for an extended period, or even permanently in some cases. Nonacting out partners don't necessarily declare a sexual moratorium, but they often employ syllogisms that yield this effect. If the sexually addicted partner is feeling deprived of sex, the impacted other might feel compassionate, but assigns the sexual need to an addictive, pathological state of mind, not the normalcy of desire: if desiring sex, then addiction. For these women, such thoughts, coupled with codependency treatment mantras like "you can't control the addict," become the pretexts for a comprehensive withdrawal from sex and, more importantly, even conversations about sex.

As a result, the impetus to resolve what may have been a long-standing sexual impasse is placed on indefinite hold, further predicated on the common belief that addiction recovery carries associations with abstinence. For those that don't install this sexual demise, safety is a legitimate concern because infidelities and prostitute-seeking behaviors place impacted partners at risk for a sexually transmitted disease or urinary tract infections. Or they might simply feel used when they do submit to sex. Understandably, they become preoccupied with their partners' preoccupation: "Who or what is he thinking about while having sex with me?" You can imagine how such a person copes with this stressor. Now, imagine the detached, "not there" sexual response of the impacted partner, which mirrors the lack of presence in the acting out figure; this "induced" state is an experience projected *into* the other.

After a spell of supposed good behavior, the designated addict tends to want credit or forgiveness. This might take tangible form as a lessening of accusations, or the return of sex, or fewer references to acting out behaviors—the "rehashing or re-opening wounds." They want a ceasefire, and there is perhaps something microcosmic in the male complaint, "I'm tired of your criticism and nagging," coupled with the female reply, "Well, you deserve it." The trouble is, *she* cannot accept that her partner is NOT acting out simply because he says so—you cannot prove a negative. Acting out a legalistic paradigm, both sides want proof, which often leads couples to polygraph examiners—ex-cops, typically, earning a second income in a niche market. Polygraph exams are sex addiction treatment's answer to the urinalysis testing of a drug treatment program, only polygraphs are more expensive. We think such exams have a one or two-instance value, because specific questions can be tailored and answered, and then a starting point for behavior change can be marked. Or not, if the person doesn't pass the exam. Aside from the expense that makes regular polygraph use available only to the wealthy, we think that it's an artificial answer to a complex question: how does a couple impacted by sex addiction rebuild trust?

Forgiveness, Mindreading, and Rebuilding Trust

And not just trust, but also mutual faith in each other through forgiveness and mutual esteem. Invoked as much by nonreligious patients as by the devout, forgiveness can seem like an oppressive gesture. It's a blessing that nonacting out partners often feel pressured to give, but resist giving cheaply. Forgiveness is a sought-after gift bestowed by the betrayed figure, but the would-be addict rarely directs this spiritual gift inwardly. Asking "When will she forgive me?" begs a self-directed counter-query: "How can you forgive yourself?" We're not suggesting that sex addicts or others who act out sexually don't merit forgiveness. Instead, we're pointing out that sex addicts shouldn't simply assign the act of forgiving to another.

While the acting out partner goes about attending groups and therapy, and seemingly not acting out (or at least not getting caught), the impacted partner waits uncertainly, observing, seeking counsel, and gauging her feelings about what is happening and what isn't. She vacillates between wanting recommitment and renewed closeness and demanding that the recovering sex addict back off, take the couch or find a hotel room. Would-be sex addicts tend to abhor emotional argument.[5] Raised to honor rationality and the presentation of evidence to judge guilt or innocence, they bristle at a therapist's privileging of feeling states over logical polemics, or the unfairness of capriciously imposed "boundaries." Some of these men welcome polygraph exams (if they are confident about passing them), hungry for an objective affirmation of their honesty and eager to give their one-and-only "I told you so" amid all the recriminations they endure. They disdain "gut instincts" and mock expectations that they "read minds" to always know what is wanted or what is felt.

Such "mindreading" is not a paranormal activity or a strictly anticipatory behavior. Instead, the term as we use it pertains to the kind of empathetic muscle necessary in all relationships. The concept of empathy is often distorted. When fielding complaints from their partners, our sex addict patients sometimes respond with, "Well, I feel like a piece of shit," thinking that this expression is empathetic because it is self-effacing and self-referential. It's not. We suggest an alternative like, "That must have been shitty for *you*," to express the salience of the other's experience in an empathetic expression.

The rebuke of mindreading as a purported subset of emotional intelligence is interesting. People seem to forget its role in their original strategies of courting, or their once-upon-a-time flirtations as fumbling teens. Who wouldn't admit that most instances of attraction were first conveyed by a quick glance or a suggestive gaze up and down another's frame rather than a finely crafted soliloquy?

---

5. We might contrast Freud's (1894) displacing, repressing obsessive with patients described by Bion (1959), whose "attacks on linking" theory described a state of mind in which emotion is hated; that a prototype object—a breast—doesn't take in (introject) and modify feeling states, which leads, paradoxically, to an intensification of feeling. It may be anyone's guess where any addicted individual fits in this neurotic-psychotic continuum.

How often do sexual invitations occur with gestures rather than words? The insistence on rationality and the hegemony of words when the context is no longer romantic seems prim. Why aren't feelings of loneliness, rejection, resentment, or fear interpreted as readily, with words so difficult to come by? Well, we know why. Sex and aggression elicit raw feelings and therefore raw expressions, so words in that context are often excused. Moreover, according to a tenet of psychoanalysis, sexual relationships are a recapitulation of early childhood development; people find in their partners some reenactment of love or intimacy that was once provided by caregivers. The wordlessness of romance seems to return us to an idealized, joyous preverbal state, while nonsexual aspects of adulthood relationships compel the strained effect of words. Regardless, nonverbal modes of expression continue their impact.

CASE ILLUSTRATION: THE RETURN OF ANNE

War trauma. Developmental trauma. Cumulative trauma. Deprivation trauma. Cultural trauma. Sexual trauma. Episodic trauma. These are just some of the terms for categories of trauma. In presenting a case that illustrates psychoanalytic therapy with a patient who has experienced episodic trauma through the discovery of sexual acting out, we operate from the premise that a more pervasive historical trauma may have preceded the patient's presenting crisis. Two types of dissociation, as outlined by Diamond (1997, 2020), may be exhibited by a patient:

1. A trance-like, thought-fragmented, or "hypnoid" state that protects against annihilation fears.
2. A less passive version may be activated in an analytic setting. It entails bringing to the surface unacceptable object representations in the transference relationship.

In this case, terms like "acting out" and splitting fade into the conceptual background. They are replaced by the similar but more nuanced concepts of dissociation, projective identification, and enactment. The patient enters treatment in the aftermath of an episodic, or "actual" trauma: the discovery of a sexual acting out pattern by an intimate partner. What the analytic therapist must do is validate the patient's experience so that secondary revisions, including insight into object relations fantasies, might occur later in the treatment process. In the meantime, the therapist must vicariously experience the traumatic anxieties, defenses, and internal object relations of the patient. By optimal absorption of this individual's pain, analytic therapists can eventually position themselves to analyze negative transferences, and, through these interventions, help the patient work through traumas that have damaged relationships over time.

> You first met Rick and Anne back in Chapter 1. After a year had passed, Anne called me, asking for an appointment. Ordinarily, after having seen a caller's partner in therapy, I would refer the caller to another clinician due to the potential confidentiality dilemma. But in her call, Anne insisted that she wanted to speak about herself and would not request any information about Rick's disclosures or my assessment of him. I reviewed the situation and considered my options. I was no longer seeing Rick in therapy, which Anne already knew. I hadn't met with him in months. His treatment had barely passed beyond the assessment phase, dwindling as episodes do sometimes, with patients canceling sessions or looking to reschedule with sketchy pretexts. The arrangement soon collapsed as Rick drifted away, bidding a half farewell with a tersely worded text. I asked Anne if it was OK for me to contact Rick, to whom she was still married, to ask him if he'd mind if I met with her. A day or so later Rick took my call, greeting me as cheerfully as if we'd spoken just a week earlier. He seemed not to care one way or another. "We pretty much live separate lives," he offered casually, stopping short of disparaging Anne as he once had, or of updating me on his progress with respect to his acting out patterns. Figuring that it was no longer my business, I did not press him. He didn't seem to know why Anne wanted therapy with me, and it didn't seem to matter to him. I pictured his demeanor and lean muscular physicality. He'd be dressed in workout attire, lifting a weight with his free arm, exercising his bicep and perhaps checking out a website for a male enhancement product as we spoke. He evinced that taut *I got this* air that alpha men like to project—right before they attempt suicide, I sometimes worry. If he was still in therapy, I'd be thinking of affect, self, and defense: a triangular framework that calls for mirroring interpretations, observing narcissistic vulnerability beneath an affectless front.

Mirroring interpretation is a technique in which a denied or split-off state of psychic pain, plus the defensive maneuver that protects against that pain, is observed by the treating professional. In Masterson's Disorder of Self model, the technique presupposes a narcissistic personality structure, a pathological term that draws attention to an intrapsychic problem of unknown pedigree, not an externalized problem. The term narcissism is pejorative to the ears of most consumers and explicit reference to such an assessment is contraindicated due to the problem of confusion. The term's connotations are critical, which unnecessarily activates a defense when access to a denied state is the indicated task. In our opinion, the offhand assignment of narcissism to sex addicts betrays unsympathetic countertransference by sex addiction specialists.

> Recall that I'd met Anne at the outset of their posttreatment (their so-called aftercare plan). And prior to that, I'd spoken to her by phone, consulting with her before meeting either of them. Intrigued, I agreed to meet her again. In the interim, they had tried couples therapy a second time, mostly to provide Anne with a full disclosure exercise. It hadn't gone well, at least not from her point of view. In the disclosure sessions, Rick was honest but not candid about his acting out history. He'd answered questions well enough when prompted but did not volunteer his former secrets as Anne expected. She complained that his disclosure wasn't good enough. He, in turn, complained that once again *he* was not good enough, like it was all a self-fulfilling prophecy.

This outcome was predictable and speaks to an important distinction between typical systemic approaches to addiction and our psychodynamic approach. A collaborative sex addiction specialist might carefully gauge the acting out person's readiness to share fully his history, but privilege an impacted partner's "right to know" and press for that forensic disclosure exercise. The impacted partner's need to know the truth, to set the broken bones of the relationship before discussing the fleshy complications, carries the moral weight in these situations. This overrules caveats by motivational interviewers, attachment specialists who warn against potential misalignments in therapy—those moments in which a clumsy therapist has failed to "back off" because that's what the patient (but not the shadow consumer) wants. It resembles an investigatory mandate sometimes heard in drug treatment programs: *must get the truth*. So, our bias is clear: people tell their shameful truths if and when they feel safe and ready to do so, not because they're supposed to.

When I met with Anne in my office she was as I'd previously remembered her: brittle, acerbic, exuding a haughty air and speaking in a clipped voice. Her face was so still that it looked as though it had absorbed a pound of Botox, yet somehow in the 1/10th of a second[6] it took for my impression to form, she evinced a warmth (or pain) that drew me in. An attractive, early middle-aged woman from a stable and loving family of origin (from her initial report), she had two children, the younger of which was on the cusp of adulthood. She was staring down the barrel of the empty nest and growing old with Rick, and was clearly depressed at the prospect, having exhausted efforts to monitor him or sustain behavior agreements. Still, I knew she wouldn't make me work the way I'd had to with Rick, who'd acted like adolescents do when they're in therapy at their parents' insistence. Anne wouldn't shrug or give monosyllabic or dull, uninterested answers, and she wouldn't simply whine that she wasn't getting credit for having behaved well since her latest atrocity. As she sat across from me, Anne spoke freely, not waiting for an inquisitive routine that she'd complain about later. Instead, she seemed eager to express herself and reflect on complicated questions. She'd gaze at me or past me, seeming to wonder what I thought but not demanding pat answers. Not anymore. She'd learned that much, it seemed, though she still held a few pat answers of her own.

Anne had tried a few things, like attending partner support groups, and had read another book or two. She interweaved comments about Rick with borrowed narratives: her

---

6. A study by Dimberg, Thunberg, and Elmehed (2000) demonstrated that adults cannot escape responding to facial emotion. In their experiment, two slides of faces with neutral poses sandwiched a slide of one face with an emotional expression; each was shown to subjects for 30 milliseconds. They found that 1/10 of a second is required for conscious recognition. While subjects reported seeing only the neutral faces in the study, facial electrodes were activated by the third, showing that they reacted to the fleeting emotional expression. So emotional reactions can be evoked out of awareness, suggesting that face-to-face communication is unconscious.

"typical" husband, who wasn't accommodating enough; who was abusive (but not violent) when he got angry; too weak to handle a strong woman when she was angry. She'd gone to a couple of female therapists since Rick had stopped working his program. Both had encouraged her to leave Rick, which she didn't want to do.

"What do you want?" I asked on cue. Her eyes rolled slightly. I could tell she was holding back stinging sarcasm as she said, "I keep asking myself that. In terms of what actions to take, I don't know. But the reason I'm back—the reason I wanted to speak to you—is because of something Rick said months ago that he attributed to you, though it paraphrases something he says from time to time, sort of." She then fell silent, leaving a pause of nearly a minute. During that time I might have shrugged, as if embodying her husband, who she said she wouldn't talk about. Apparently, a remark of his was the pretext for this next episode. I took note of the feeling, an inducement from afar. Rick was like a ghost. He'd have bailed from one of my groups had I admitted him, which is why I didn't. Now, I was perhaps finally getting this taste of his feelings: tension or dread or former excitement that he wanted no part of anymore. At the same time, I felt for Anne, who likely felt his excitement once, only to lose that feeling. I wanted to know what this thing was that I'd supposedly said or drawn from Rick. She *candidly* volunteered it: "He said that you said that I had to deal with my part of the problem, which reminded me that he always used to complain, 'you never look at your part,' which he never explains, or can't. Well, I remember talking to you nearly a year ago, on the phone and then in here. I remember you talking about how important it was to try and understand the problem from all sides and not just . . . something like that. I don't know. I didn't really like the message at the time. It sounded wishy-washy yet blaming. Anyway, I want to understand what my part is, whatever that means."

Wishy-washy yet blaming. I'm sure my feedback would have sounded that way. I contemplated Anne's need to devalue me ahead of therapy, preempting some anticipated counter-criticism. Although she bristled at the frequency, Anne and I started meeting twice per week to talk about her *part* in a broken marriage, plus the OR "system" from which she had emerged.

That expression—*what's your part?*—is one we've been hearing for years in the context of drug or sex addiction treatment. It's an interesting euphemism intended to reduce or alter constructs of responsibility or blame to abstractions with elusive or secretive meanings. Its purpose is to inject space for a consideration of roles. The word "part" seems like a synonym for psychological casting, a phenomenon shrouded in a modern, as yet undefined taboo: *don't go there*. Such an interpretation could lead partners like Anne back to square one, to thinking of herself in more recognizable terms such as "victim" or its more empowering relative, "survivor."

> Anne hadn't lasted long in her women's support groups because she didn't like the nomenclature. She especially disliked the term *victim*, but not because she rejected evidence to support use of the word. Indeed, when she considered all of the reasons Rick might have acted sexually outside of their marriage, she couldn't think of one that was anything close to her fault. "Not really," she added cautiously.
>
> Something was nagging at her. It wasn't enough for her to segregate her life from Rick in various ways, like practicing self-care (taking time away to go on short vacations with girlfriends), or demanding that he take vacations, meaning impromptu overnights to anywhere else—to the doghouse, as Rick had said. As far as she was concerned, she had already separated psychologically by increasing attention to her own career, focusing on her kids, and maintaining friendships with one or two confidantes from her college years. She did not want to reconcile fully with her husband. She'd long since wearied of Rick's workaholic, alcoholic, and now sex addict (sexaholic?) patterns, all of which congealed around a singular idea: he didn't want to deal with life, or people. He might not want to deal with her specifically, but the observation that he avoided people generally seemed to deflect from this other, more hurtful point. That observation distilled at least one challenging question: why was she with him? Or why had she attached her life to his in the first place? It seemed unlikely that he'd been so different when they'd first met in their 20s.
>
> Over multiple sessions, Anne continued her habit of impugning Rick whenever she mentioned him. Occasionally she'd complain, wondering why I wasn't stopping her from talking about him, since figuring out "her part" was

the ostensible goal of her treatment. I pointed out that I'd observed her focus on Rick numerous times, only for her to argue the point. "I'm expressing my feelings," she would say, to which I would reply, "no, you're representing him and sticking the words 'I feel' in front of your thought." Her contradiction made her resistance apparent: she pretended to share responsibility, but her habit betrayed her wish to have no demands placed on her. I offered that she wanted me to stop her complaining to protect her from the discomfort of exposure. She didn't like her angry self, I constructed, treading on tender ground. More than once she scoffed at this suggestion. In fact, she repeatedly denied my observations of defenses despite asking me to look at them.

After such exchanges Anne apologized, thinking herself ungrateful in challenging my approach and insights. After all, I was listening to her, which is what I'd promised I'd do more than anything; it was one of many things Rick didn't do. He didn't do apologies (though Rick insisted he had, ad nauseam). He didn't do empathy. He wouldn't listen. "I did so much. He did so little!" she exclaimed, referring to a variety of his failings, the least of which pertained to sex. This was interesting, as his sexual betrayal of her was the only complaint that I had explicitly validated. It now seemed that she expected more from me.

As she did most of the talking in sessions, I soon perceived transference in her remarks. She seemed needful yet Bovarist, opportunistic, and at times manipulative. She wasn't as selfless as she thought she was. The more I let her speak, the more I supplied the rope with which she might hang herself. She couldn't stop devaluing Rick, as if it were a compulsion. She also couldn't stop baiting me to play the disapproving patriarch who would blame her and assign her a "part" that would render her culpable for what was in his nature (*I didn't make him eat the apple!*). Or maybe I'd think her unreasonable or too angry—a *bitch*. In stepping into this projection, I was supposed to exhibit weariness about her complaints and then criticize her attitude. In so doing, I would demonstrate that I couldn't deal with her, enabling her avoidance of truth. In an effort to not play my part, I threw a wrench into the works, and began to confront the falseness of her protests:

"Sounds like you tolerated how he was."

"I didn't," she responded, looking confused by my supposition. "Wait, what do you mean?"

"Sounds like you stopped having expectations of him. You judge him—put him down, I hear—but you're only critical. You don't hold him to expectations. You let go, give up."

She sighed, conceded my point, then moved to justify herself. She said that it wouldn't work to protest continually. Besides, they'd simply fight afterward.

"How was that?" I asked.

"Horrible," she replied. "He can hurt me. I can hurt him." She couldn't—or wouldn't—say how they hurt each other. Perhaps she couldn't remember, or maybe she didn't want to think about it. When asked to recall the hurtful words, Anne backslid, became disorganized and vague, and said "I don't know" repeatedly, retreating much like Mr. A (the stolid patient illustrated in Chapter 1), though her retreat seemed closer to her mind's surface.

After an hour like this, she'd cancel the next session. Although it did not invoke the trauma of her recent or distant past, she'd excuse herself from the process, claiming to need a break from treatment. Taking a break like this, or a vacation, is another of Western society's paradigmatic beliefs. It allows people to seek respite without disturbing inertia. On her return I confronted the avoidance by interpreting its self-protective function. Pain was emerging, but she was as adept as an addict at nipping it in the bud. That said, I didn't need to compare her to an addict to witness her fragility. I perceived her defense. She seemed angry and sought to bully away my observations, casting my insights as formulaic and banal. I was almost as bad as Rick, she insinuated. God forbid an experienced, licensed professional therapist would ever lack empathy, I reminisced.

An intermittent stalemate persisted for months before anything broke. Then, during a session in which I was feeling sluggish and absent, she again pointed out that she was doing almost all of the talking—the lion's share of the work, as she thought of it. Feeling defensive and thinking that I was failing as an object, I offered her a clumsy yet serendipitous question: "Why is my talking so important?" This made her angry. Initially, she smiled, then looked away and dipped her hand into her purse in search of an item. For a moment, it looked like the kind of gesture a woman might make just before leaving a restaurant table, disgusted by an obnoxious or absent-minded date. I said nothing as she plucked a hand-held mirror from her bag, held it to her face, and inspected her eyes.

"What's happening?" I asked evenly.

"I don't know, thought I'd . . . thought you were going to say something else. That's all."

"Something you hoped I'd say, perhaps?"

She smiled again, a bit derisively, like she was putting me in my place (whatever that place now was). She asked me a question: "Does your . . . technique, style, or whatever, ever include what you might think of as encouragement, or reassurance, or validation? You don't seem to do much of that." Glancing at my degree and license certificates, she seemed poised to attack my credentials and take aim at my ego. She sighed and looked away again as I began to formulate what was happening.

I replied: "Your comment suggests you want more but you've stopped."

She glared at me. Thinking it was rage, I briefly wanted out of the room. This would have been the point at which Rick would leave, thinking he'd escape being struck by a flying object or a piercing remark.

"I'm sorry. I didn't mean to be rude. Not the first time for that, I'm sure," she said, the heat still in her eyes.

I was ready to confront this statement, ask her why she owed me an apology, or suggest its falseness in some way. "I understand that you're sorry, yet you still seem angry, and the apology doesn't extinguish that, I think. I get the feeling you're holding back, retreating again from your feelings, and perhaps concerned about what might happen if you truly express what you want."

"I don't want to say something I'd regret," she said icily, as if I was placing her in a bind and asking too much of her. Then her tone softened. "You've been kind and patient, and listening, and . . ." she trailed off.

"Have I? Sounds like you thought me anything but kind, patient, and listening a few moments ago. What changed? You seemed angry, perhaps hurt when I questioned the importance of my talking. Then you made an apology and started complimenting me, as if the anger was a problem." In a sense, I was admitting to letting her down, not because that was material or objective reality, but instead because it reflected the psychic reality of Anne's experience, present and past.

It was during this (edited but real) exchange that the associations began to flow, stirred by an exchange she'd had with Rick that recalled elements of our sessions.

"It was weird, he just lost it," she began, relating an altercation that had been triggered by a seeming triviality. The "it" in her expression was actually a useful metaphor, even though the dispute had been about something else. The misplacement of an item symbolized displacement from the couple's chronic turmoil. She and Rick had been in their car, about to enter the driveway of their home, only to have their approach thwarted because the garage door opener (the "clicker") was not in its usual place below the dashboard. A petty squabble ensued and then escalated, with each partner digging their heels in and showing their spots. Anne insisted that Rick's wayward mind—his inattention to detail and the needs of others—was the true culprit. Rick was defiant, but she was convinced that the clicker had been mislaid by him.

Wrong. Two days later, the item was found by a housekeeper, lodged in a bag that belonged to Anne. The evidence was irrefutable: Anne had dropped the clicker in her bag and either hadn't noticed it or had forgotten about it. Unfortunately—or not—the housekeeper's discovery happened live, in front of the couple after Anne had asked her to check the bag for something else while they were all together in the kitchen. "What's this?" the woman asked innocently, raising the clicker aloft, not knowing the meaning of her discovery. Anne strode toward the hapless woman, snatching the clicker away like it was a toy being held by a recalcitrant child. Sheepish, she avoided eye contact with Rick, but offered him a smile moments after dismissing the housekeeper from the room. She was embarrassed but, for the moment, more in touch with her amusement. Rick didn't share in the lighthearted spirit and stiffly demanded an apology. She tried to brush it off, seeing the funny side and wanting him to see it too. She did eventually make amends, but not with the straight-faced solemnity that Rick seemed to want. Her flippancy triggered rage in Rick, who then stormed out of the room, hurling insults and profanity. They'd barely spoken since.

"What did he want me to say?" she asked at the session. I remained silent, as I often do when a patient speaks at length on a subject and then asks me to analyze someone not in the room. The session proceeded brokenly, with Anne offering bits and pieces. She wanted me to respond, to do this creative work for her. The expression in her eyes and the tightness of her voice seemed to say, "Don't just sit there and listen." I could have asked her to wonder aloud what was on Rick's mind, what he may have wanted her to say, what his nonsexual needs were in that moment. I held off on these questions, and for the moment I focused on her process, that curious movement from caught red-handed exposure to embarrassment, to irritable gesture, to laughing escape. What had been on her mind? And what did *she* want? Not surprisingly, she wanted those aforementioned feelings to go away, so she orated her way through them, drawing conclusions and writing a script I couldn't possibly contest. I recalled the dialogue between that couple presented earlier—"he's careless with things and therefore us"—plus other spikes of shame stirred by common wrongdoings, like being wrong about a missing clicker.

"I get that I was in the wrong this time," she said finally, and reluctantly. "But don't you think he should get over it? I have to get over all of his shit." By implication, his shit was a lot worse; their complaints to each other were asymmetrical. By this point, Anne was looking away, having grown accustomed to me not answering her leading questions.

Her pause had left space for me to respond. "Well, the question is what is there to get over? What might be clicking?"

"What?" Anne responded.

I clarified. "This incident with the clicker seems to have stirred something important, an upset that isn't resolved."

Her expression flattened as she facetiously said something about not expecting answers to her questions, especially those about people not in the room. I guess I'd used that phrase before, so now she was throwing it in my face. I replied that she seemed plaintive, but was couching her protest in passive terms and holding resentment toward me. She interrupted my trailing words, asking, "What am I supposed to say?" which mirrored the complaint she aimed at Rick and suggested a bind.

I stuttered. "I'm . . . not sure what you want me to say." After a few stumbling, awkward moments, which were also checkered with stop-start utterances on her part, I continued. I utilized my idea of an evidence-based approach, referencing the words—her words—that constructed either her conscious intentions, or her unconscious purpose: "You've indicated that you were in the wrong on this occasion, but that he overreacted to your error with the clicker, and demanded an apology. More broadly, you've asked me to reflect back to you on what your part is in conflicts. Well, what you tend to report are stories of Rick's wrongdoings, which are numerous and hurtful. However, when something is your fault, as in the clicker anecdote, you offer a brief recognition of your wrongdoing, followed by a quick refocus on Rick, plus a tacit expectation that I validate this response, and the narrative that his few legitimate complaints are trivial while yours are important. Or—and sometimes this happens in here, with me—you apologize for what you think is your rudeness, but more to hide your anger or prevent doing harm, rather than say fully what you think, or feel, or want. These, I think, are examples of your part."

She opened her mouth but didn't speak. Instead, she vocalized something that could have been helplessness, or disorientation.

"I don't know what to do with that," she finally complained, flustered.

"Well, before deciding what to do, what do you think about what I've said?" At this she floundered again, so I tried something less heady, more of a dive into transference: "You see, I think something happens when you and I speak of these things. I think you want some manner of caring, like acknowledgment from me of how awful things are for you, and when I don't offer it, or don't offer it enough, you feel not only criticized, but unfairly treated, and then I seem uncaring to you. And if this is your lot in life then you're left with feeling bad about that or else striking out with anger, which might feel worse. Maybe you're not sure what you deserve."

For subsequent sessions, I offered an arrangement of three meetings per week, which Anne accepted. There were more enactments and more instances of transference acting out—meaning, resistances to the therapeutic relationship. That's the nature of intensive, ongoing treatment. Character traits reveal themselves repeatedly in the office space, which heightens the resistance of patients who can't just run out the clock as they might during short-term programs. Eventually, Anne stopped acting out, instead turning her thoughts to the manner and history of her fighting, as well as its part in a paradoxical habit of avoidance.

Having once given a tidy, curated version of her family history, she later associated toward memories of difficult parents and competitive, bickering siblings, and linked these associations to her reactions in treatment. Her parents were preoccupied with their careers, although her mother had reduced hers somewhat in deference to her husband's working life. It was hard getting either of them to listen. Dad was often absent; even when he was present, he seemed uninterested. Mom was uninterested also, but more directly critical of Anne, often shushing her when she talked too much. Eventually, it seems that Anne compensated by cajoling, and later bullying, with her own criticisms.

She observed everyone's "unloving" ways, identifying with her mother and regaining lost feelings of infantile omnipotence, but also identifying her father's aggression with her *ferocity*. She described her history with a quaver in her voice, like she was clinging to a shaken foundation. She once thought that if she was capable and compliant, or if she listened to others and reflected them, they would surely reciprocate. She hadn't accounted for the insatiability of others or her own capacity for rage, which she still denied, though it continued to peek above the surface. Her hopeful interest in others later turned to lecturing and attacking instead of listening, and discharging her rage while maintaining that she was loving. "I'm trying to help," she'd defend, hoping she deserved to be loved in return. She also hedged her bets. If she was perfect, or self-sufficient, it would block her need for others' love.

"I don't know if they like me, let alone love me. I don't know if anyone likes me, if you like me."

With Rick she reenacted much of this history—perhaps her own narcissistic wound. Though she stopped short of making that link, Rick likely resembled her father, with whom she'd unconsciously bonded by finding in Rick a like replacement, at least originally. This is the ego's compromise: it has "lost" the object, which induces melancholia, but it is not "given up" if the primal attachment is reenacted. Rick and Anne were once competent flirts and kindred spirits: they were both athletic, physically attractive, ambitious, and hard-working, and neither suffered fools gladly. They loved each other's confidence and independence. They wouldn't need each other, so they didn't take care, and problems within this false contract began to mount. Careers and child-rearing furthered their distance, creating pretext after pretext for ignoring each other's denied needs. Among friends and family, date nights and "quality time" were duly and laughingly referenced as antidotes to the querulous inquiry, "Who has the time to relax these days?" But the loneliness was real, and the coping strategy was derivative.

Rick manifested a grim, sacrificial, resentment-building false self that split off needs for nurturing and attached them to novelty and transience within a flood of alcohol consumption. He may have enacted what is often presumed to be the male (and therefore most commonly known) version of the Oedipal task: identify with the father, whether he is a decent, law-abiding citizen, a hyper-libidinous aggressor, or something in between. Taking possession of and subduing women, or looking to identify with their positive qualities (the Jungian observation of the anima), represented attempts to recover what he had lost but not given up. To Rick, Anne may have represented some messy blend of his mother's good and bad, and it wasn't long before the bad seemed to overtake the good, as far as he was concerned. Anne tried to change him, boss him, and "help" him, hoping he'd notice her needs as a reward. However, he did not notice her needs in the way analytic therapy did, which evoked the pain of awareness. When the intimacy she sought was not forthcoming, her dam broke, unleashing her bitterness about his failures with respect to money management; his dismissive, careless attitude toward their children, especially their daughter; and his regular impotence, which she took personally and found humiliating. Climactically, she goaded him with an antiquated put-down that persists in the postfeminist era: "You're not a real man."

> As Anne recounted how she had lashed out and attacked Rick, both before and after discovery of his acting out, she pieced together the part she'd played—her cruel streak. She was a hurt, angry woman. I listened in a way that acknowledged the legitimacy of her anger. However, it also stirred anxiety; she couldn't trust that someone might care for her and believe that she was important while maintaining that she wasn't always right. She habitually defended by externalizing with cold rage, which would bully others into a retreat that would confirm her view of herself as "unimportant." Despite my challenging (and at times skeptical) air, she took me in, accepting that I cared. I found myself having to manage a fear that I'd absorbed (PI) from her as well as (indirectly) from Rick: a fear of not measuring up. During our sessions, we didn't talk that much about sex. It didn't *flow* easily, suggesting blocked erotic transference, or social/gender barriers that psychoanalysts strain to navigate.
>
> I've presented Rick and Anne in bookending fashion because I find them typical of the male and female partners who present for care in the context of sex addiction treatment. Rick was a dismissive, avoidantly attached male, likely addicted but nonetheless acting out split-off feeling states. Anne was an ambivalently attached woman who was relationally preoccupied but also distancing.

The pathology of such couples, of impacted partners, or of FSLAs, probably bears more study. But we think there's a problem: Mental health researchers often comment that feminine psychology is understudied. If this is true, maybe it's because contemporary discussion invariably circles back to pathologies assigned to men or limits imposed by male society. For example, narcissism is diagnosed in both men and women, but a passing glance at cultural trends suggests that narcissism is a dominantly male condition, though we believe this prejudice is far less pronounced among analytic thinkers. Women more often get assigned personality traits (like Borderline Personality Disorder) that are virtually synonymous with trauma, so even the diagnosis of BPD is a backhanded swipe at society. Many speak pejoratively of the masculine gaze, but what do we think of the feminine swoon? Is swooning even a problem? If so, what age-old story does it tell? The Madonna-whore complex is commonly known by lay readers as a concept that denotes men's capacity for splitting the feminine image. What do we suppose women direct at men, leading them to inhabit harmful dichotomies? Be a badass at work, then bulk up at the gym; but then come home, calm down, help make a meal, then put the kids to bed or fix the air conditioning unit but don't explain how you fixed the air conditioning unit. Later, enfold your woman into your brawny chest and listen to what her day was like. Perhaps she'll laud you for a deft straddling of the hero/strength-vulnerability split with no catchy mythical name (incidentally, "knight in shining armor" references an idealized pole, not the split).

> What did Anne want from Rick? She identified as a feminist, claiming a desire to play, bond, and partner with a man who could access vulnerability but otherwise be strong. Did she welcome his vulnerability? Ultimately, Anne admitted that her declining interest in their sex life had predated discovery of Rick's acting out, and that his mid-life loss of confidence—his "weakness"—was a turn-off.

Anne is not unique. Many women seem progressive but actually disdain vulnerability in men, whether it is acted out, defended against with grandiosity, or expressed humbly with words and beseeching tears. What such women seem to want from men is an unknown chimera drawn from lost mythology, or a mythopoeic phenomenon as yet unnamed, though we can ourselves formulate, imagine, and think about the altered state of masculine ego.

Let's imagine that the knight is analogous to the whore. Why the whore? Historically, men are desired and exploited for their violent capacities or heroic aspirations, so the knight is to violence and sacrifice what the whore is to sex. Unlike the whore, the knight is often (but not always) revered for playing that role, but he frequently dies, is maimed, or is defeated for the sake of placating or arousing women. What corresponds to the Madonna? A saint? A priest? A therapist, doctor, brother, or father who deliberately rejects the knight role, privately burning today's more variable draft cards? Are these figures sexy, as reflected in the mythos of our times, and should young men aspire to their qualities, thinking a lean in that direction is both socially just and in their sexual interests? Or do such men risk becoming "soft males," as Bly (1990) put it, destined to be rejected by women who are as conflicted in their desires as men are in theirs? Or, as men like Rick might ask, is there any winning with them?

We understand the progressive intellectual's fear of an antifeminist backlash.[7] Contemporary rhetoric volleys accusations of "false equivalency" and "hypocrisy" as thought vetoes, reflecting tussles over righteousness and sexual and economic freedom, with leftover rewards of shame and guilt reduction. We understand that this is an era of payback, or justice (a nobler term), so men like Rick aren't meant to be "winning" and we know that cutting slack on today's corsets is *de rigueur* while the leash on Rover is tightened. Overall, we think that these are the reasons that female sex addiction or the plight of impacted partners is less often studied or treated, not the nonsense that fewer resources are available for afflicted women. Protestations about the allocation of resources reflect beliefs about feminine disadvantage, which is now a cultural tautology. However, there are plenty of capable therapists, male and—especially—female, who are willing to talk to women about sex and addiction, whether they speak in bumper sticker platitudes or, more interestingly, find ways to penetrate minds with care.

> The postscript to the case of Rick and Anne is not a happy one, but it was not a straightforward rupture or a confirmation of Rick's defeatism. Unsurprisingly, they did not resume couples therapy. It was unclear whether Rick ceased his once acknowledged acting out pattern. He'd long since punted on their marriage, so he was unprepared for Anne's modest, ambiguous contrition. After a while, she relayed to him the substance of our sessions, and in particular her inventory

7. Gilligan (2010) argued that by placing the Oedipal myth at the center of psychoanalysis, Freud disavowed the voices of women who claimed sexual trauma, instead submitting to patriarchal culture and casting women as secretive and difficult while privileging his own fantasies of an incestuous relationship with his mother. Biblical, Arthurian, Norse, Chinese, Egyptian, Indonesian, Japanese, and Greek mythologies all feature examples of the incest taboo, with some indicating mother-son incest (e.g., the Greek myth of Titan parents Gaia and Uranus). It might alternatively be suggested that Freud "privileged" a myth that ultimately maligns masculine fantasy, that he proposed transcendence to indulgence of the wish. It's interesting to note that in the Oedipal myth, Oedipus's mother, Jocasta, is a figure of mystery: did she support her husband Laius in leaving the child Oedipus to die so that he wouldn't grow up to kill his father (the oracle's prophecy that stirs the drama), or did she secretly give the child to a shepherd to be rescued and raised separately by the king and queen of Corinth?

of "lashings-out" that she'd directed at him over years. She conceded that sometimes she was wrong or overreacted. At other times she underreacted, like he did, to block how much their estrangement hurt her. Anne reported that Rick was moved by this gesture and became somewhat more considerate. Her gesture was part begrudging concession and part painful admission; she otherwise maintained that Rick was still 90% to blame for their problems. Or maybe 75%, she amended with a coy smile, by then defending with mischief and less menace. Today, Anne and Rick remain together as a couple, living some manner of homeostasis while Anne tolerates him—and herself—just a little bit more.

CHAPTER 5

Sex Addiction and Group Therapy

> I refuse to join any club that would have me as a member.
>
> —Groucho Marx

It's difficult enough thinking by yourself. It's even more difficult to think in a one-on-one interaction, or within the triangle of couples therapy. Then there's thinking in a group. Yet we as individuals are asked by society to think in groups, as a part of something bigger, whether we like it or not, because the group is where morals, ethics, rules, and meaning are really made. This is not an idle, essayist opinion (though it is idly borrowed from Immanuel Kant). We have facilitated therapy groups for 25 years—a long time to be doing something wrong, someone once quipped—and at any given time within that stretch, belonging to a group, or feeling separate from groups, has seemed crucial. Yet, in this sheltered, introverted COVID moment of 2020 and into 2022, our sense of group identity, group participation, and inclusion (or exclusion) feels amplified. The tension between individualism versus collective need has been thrust center stage, with the former principled position threatened in the light of social movements, the specter of a public health crisis. Indeed, many believe a problem is only a problem if it affects a group. Some clamor for the microphone. Most recede into the background or call for a pax in which commonalities override differences, helping us ignore them. We're meant to have difficult conversations live, but the topical habit is to complain about differences online, from a laptop or smartphone, in 150 characters or less. Hardly anyone seems to attend a therapy group to talk about their differences. The group's the thing, as the saying goes, where people can talk about their problems. Finding the like-minded—and remaining so—is both desired and presumed.

Freud (1921) observed that individuals lose themselves in groups, and seek illusions of leadership, hypnotic experience. Bion (1961a) expanded this vision and cast group experience as a regression, with individuals seeking leaders or pairings rather than finding their own voice. Sex addiction treatment groups aren't any different. Here's a profile of some participants:

- Men raised on the passed-down wisdom of Dale Carnegie and Marshall Field are all about drive, success, and discipline, and love saying how things are in a world that they dominate. They subdue these qualities somewhat in groups under the weight of shame, becoming reason-seeking, Saturnian figures who can charm their way out of dick-pic discoveries but not sustain a reliable presence at close quarters. They enter groups with studied urbanity, averting imagined eyes scrutinizing their characters. They privilege rationality and are prone to literalism; to them, the only digestible meaning of "act out" is a sexual act.
- Another type of group member—somewhat more hapless than the first—does a lot of shrugging, deferring to his wife's opinions about what constitutes true emotional intimacy because . . . well, because he's spent a lot less time reading about the subject, that's why. Instead, he's got his eye on the basement where that air-conditioning unit still needs fixing, and as he cedes the moral and spiritual high ground to his well-read and therapy-journeyed partner, he may wonder why he keeps agreeing to have the kitchen redone in Terra Cotta.

Notwithstanding "difficult men," we find that men will speak of sex addiction, take responsibility, and—over time—get real (honest and open-minded) in a group atmosphere that isn't hateful, pedantic, or officious. They arrive in our unlikely sanctuaries having lost themselves, but in group they find a weekly two-hour home. This belief reflects the influence of the nearly 100-year-old 12-step movement, for only addiction problems are prescribed group therapies so consistently. Because isolation seems so complicit in addiction, fellowship is a standard antidote. In addition, the group format is the closest thing psychotherapy has to creating a bridge to public opinion (as referenced in Chapter 2). So men sit in egalitarian circles and talk about sex, fantasy, and porn. Okay, they may start a group session chatting about sports, partly because they can be competitive within that context and express I HATE YOU in a contained and coded fashion. If they're feeling brave, they may talk about impotence. Or they may debate the ethics of prostitution, whether it truly demeans women or merely provides an income opportunity—sexual and economic freedom rather than slavery. However, the men we speak to aren't typically concerned with the plight of women or public morality. Individualist in spirit, they speak of their families as extensions of themselves,[1] expressing a commitment to family but not necessarily to community, much less to a group. They juxtapose fears of inclusion and exclusion, seeking to fit in while denying the importance of that very desire.

If a group's setting and atmosphere can provide the security (privacy) of a medieval keep, a therapy group can proceed with its main tasks: to discuss and rediscuss sex, support the reduction of acting out behaviors, and dull the buzz of sexual misbehavior. This pleasure buzz interferes not so much with logic as with thinking reflectively about feeling states. In groups such displays are multiplied because obsessive thinking is fixed, repetitive, inflexible, and stifles feeling. As Freud observed, feeling and reflective thought are blocked, topographically, in the unconscious and then denied entry into the conscious realm. This primary repression may explain why obsessives don't dream, or don't recall their dreams, at least. However, sensations and agitations poke through the barriers between the mental spheres, leading to suppressive action and what is termed repression proper (Freud, 1915). Consider the following illustration of thought that doesn't emerge versus thought that does and becomes available for scrutiny:

Patient 1: I didn't think of it. . . . I've no idea what happened. I just did it.

Patient 2: Well, the question came to me—should I? and I thought, sure . . . why not!

---

1. In the dawning of COVID-19, nature's most fearful predator is a virus. In their limit-setting, reality-testing role, group members caution one another that direct contact sexual acting out, especially with transient partners, is dangerous to self, but more importantly, to family and children. This latter, "unbearable" prospect suggests that a past—and still present—danger, the contagion of STDs between partners, is not so unbearable.

Patient 1 is spared the discomfort of his choice until after it's made. In contrast, Patient 2 has at least given himself something to weigh and then dismiss. Like other obsessives, Patient 2 may prefer to think about plans, machinate over minutiae, and get lost in the bells and whistles. Ultimately, if this internal habit doesn't change, it may not matter if physical, observable "acting out" ceases. Some patients lock themselves in persecutory anxiety, aping a crude notion of legal systems. Consciousness and premeditation incur harsher punishment, but "not thinking" obscures responsibility and will mitigate others' judgments. It's a risky fallacy, roughly akin to "dry drunk" thinking (as termed in AA, to indicate distortions), especially if the cessation of "actual" acting out is only a hiatus.

A Problem of Thinking: Internal Process and Defenses in Group Therapy

Shame-faced sex addicts don't share as much of their behavioral ephemera as, say, drug addicts do. Why? Sharing focuses on actions, but obsession does not preclude fear of judgment. Therefore, group members tend to spare one another what they call the "gory details," instead revealing themselves with unconscious slips and euphemisms, like "going in the back-door" in describing an affair. Later, the person using this phrase might reveal a preference for—and then an obsession with—anal sex, alongside a generalized social inhibition, layering their fear of front doors. Group members might ask, "What were you thinking?" of someone who is describing fathomless bad decisions, or "What are you thinking?" with respect to the here and now, or even "What were you feeling?" with respect to past moments.

Psychiatrist Siegel (1999) echoed psychoanalytic theory, observing that a person doesn't know their feelings in the past and they might not know their feelings in the present unless feeling states are tied to consciousness. That said, back and forth questions in a group carry a parenthetical corollary that might sound like, "Why weren't you thinking of . . .?" in reference to a foreseeable consequence of acting out such as the impact of discovery on a significant other. A person being questioned may acknowledge wrongdoing and the "valid" admonishments of the group. Focus then shifts to the decision's aftermath, the dutiful hand-wringing of guilt, which a group may defend against with supportive phrases like "don't beat up on yourself." Such exchanges reflect the "shoulds" of the group superego that bonded, committed members might dispense with over time. This doesn't mean that acting out should be condoned or that supportive gestures would be proscribed. It means only that members might become more honest about their secret rationales for acting out, such as giving up on self and others (like partners) or the tacit belief that acting out is adaptive if an ideal sex life seems unavailable. As denial and pretense subside, a group might acknowledge that inhibition of intimacy is less a "negative consequence" than a clandestine goal serving old complexes.

Disturbed by such revelations, group focus often returns to the concrete, perhaps confused by a therapeutic mantra: yes, the problem is about sex, but it's not just about sex. In analytic terms, sex breeds obsession and is a root of neurosis. However, particular sexual behaviors (perversions) serve as displacements of anxiety (which are about sex), as well as attached meanings about self and others. For example, group members tend to agree that obsessive perfection-seeking via porn use disrupts intimacy in a primary relationship because most partners cannot measure up to the ideals sought online. Evidence includes conjuring images of those fantasy figures during sex with a primary partner. Such fantasies might even happen during a group session. Indeed, some have admitted this at times, claiming to be lost or bored by group process. A female colleague who leads men's groups once said that she likes to ask the question, "How many of you are objectifying me right now?" Although we observe transference in a group setting, we're less inclined to ask this question because the "objectifying" term is too provocative among men of presumed heterosexual orientation. Instead, we phrase questions about members' responses to material more generically, at least initially: "What's the group's response? How are individuals feeling?" Group members often defend with behavioral suggestions, or by directing clarifying questions at one another in the form of probing if friendly investigations, as if trying to solve a puzzle: "How can we stop 'it' from happening again?" Despite the fear of such a process elsewhere, the process becomes a forensic exercise because the group is a "safe" space. However, questions about internal responses must be asked if another level of sharing is to occur. Associations may follow: members accustomed to process norms will offer what they think "relates" to the share of the other. In this way, members are indeed bonding by demonstrating nonjudgment and cohesion.

An interpersonal meaning may be apparent, or even conspicuous, but not readily spoken about in a group. The voice of a man who experiences a group's skepticism may rise defensively as he answers questions. If his inquisitors don't notice and continue to engage on a Socratic level, it becomes necessary to ask, "How do you feel about X's comment?" or say, "You seemed disturbed by one or two of the others' questions." This approach is not exclusive of concrete inquiries into behavior or facts, but it seeks to integrate those efforts with an equally important process: attention to affective responses, revealing tacit messages about interdependence.

> A man anticipating a divorce considers whether he would be deterred from acting out when his marriage is officially over. Group feedback tosses around the pros and cons of the sharing member's decision, with some wondering what he is waiting for. Why wait? The discussion is broken transiently by a member who states that, while he may once have been inclined to act out if living the circumstances of his peers, over time he has come to feel an increasing obligation to the other men in the group. He might be "letting guys down" if he acts out. I have to reference his comment twice before anyone else gives the idea serious thought: would they feel guilt or shame if reporting an acting out episode to a group of men they've come to know well, and whose difficulties they share?

Do members feel a sense of responsibility to one another? A sense of community? Do they worry about being judged, still, by other men? It's remarkable how slowly and reluctantly a group responds to comments that allude to group inclusion, as if they threaten to unearth needs that have long since become dissociated.

> A member mentions visiting former sites of acting out, only to not partake in a physical act. He is proud to have "not acted out" in his (SAA) inner circle and is duly congratulated by group members. His so-called middle circle behavior was a tour of an old playground, only with a melancholic rather than excitable air. When he is asked what helped him avoid his inner circle (actually entering one of the establishments and using a service), he says, "I want to honor the people who care about me." To a man, each member

replies to this seemingly ambiguous comment with an assumption that non-group members only—the man's wife, his individual therapist, or perhaps his group therapist (me)—are the caring people in question, not them. Eventually, I pry open the in-the-moment meaning of the man's comment, which he obligingly confirms. His comment, to everyone's surprise, is aimed at the group.

Group Needs, Community Virtues

Gratitude, honoring, obligation: these are the virtuous gifts of a group process. They reflect principles of altruism and universality that are meant to underlie a group's purpose (Yalom, 1995), because group is, basically, society. Sex addiction, with its baggage of shame and guilt, adds tacit dimensions to a group's agenda, such as taming patterns of destructive behavior via self-reporting. Furthering obligation, an addiction therapy group absorbs some of the expectations of impacted parties, invisible members of the group with agendas that mimic parenting. Meanwhile, the group acts as a surrogate limit-setter, conscience, or memory system. Given sensitivities toward being controlled or lectured, members resist playing these roles directly. Imagining reciprocity, or "payback," they fear that others will assume such roles toward them. Even tentative statements in this vein are prefaced with careful disclaimers. "I'm not one to talk," a member might say if daring to confront the unmotivated attitude of a troubled peer. So-called honesty agreements, signed with spouses at the outset of treatment, can be a problem if they render some group members reticent, thinking that a group leader is obliged to inform about acting out episodes. Such agreements can diminish cohesiveness, making the group reluctant to take risks and share candidly. Echoing Bion (1961a), members look to a leader to carry the weight and spare individuals from tasks they feel disqualified from performing. In the spirit of altruism, they may find it more comfortable to recall the goals, statements, and histories of fellow members. As a result, "Didn't you tell us . . .?" moments are somewhat common in a developing group. Such questions act as a guardrail against the habit of forgetting.

However, that duty pales in comparison to asserting one's non-sexual needs. Recalling Carnes's (1991) derivative assertion that a sex addict transfers his emotional needs towards sexual acting out, we regularly observe that sex addicts struggle with the interpersonal aspects of therapy, perhaps reflecting a disordered intrapsychic structure discussed elsewhere in this text (Chapters 1 and 3). In a group, this process manifests as members assert and yield space for sharing. Often, they seem thinly aware of their interpersonal needs, such as being listened to, being heard and understood, being admired, or being cared for with suggestions or interpretations. Working on such unrecognized needs is only possible if the structure of the group allows self-activation. In other words, in a tightly structured group, with a leader who designates understood allotments of time for each member's share, there is no need for an individual to assert a need to share. The structure of this group, which reflects an artificial reality, spares individuals from that anxiety-provoking task. In contrast, in a group with an organic structure, members' latent anxieties about having their needs met are more realistically tested, for in relationships, as in life in general, there are no such guarantees.

In active discussions, the jostling for position, plus the seizing of space in which to comment or begin a share, can be competitive and stressful. A timid member may wait for minutes or sometimes over an hour before taking his opportunity to weigh in on a topic, allowing it to pass him by as he waits for an opening. One member compared the task of entering group-speak to waiting by the side of a road, aiming for an opening to cross a busy street. But the street in question is a freeway, and there are no traffic lights. This exaggeration points to the anxiety some feel when speaking in groups, especially when exposing their thoughts on the most difficult of subjects—sex—or any other topic (though sex is the constant subtext). Even more difficult than the subject is the challenge of competing for space. Once in a while, a group member takes aggressive measures to make his voice heard. He might nudge his way in or silence others. In one instance, a visibly uncomfortable member waiting for his turn eventually turned to a garrulous peer and said, "Now you've said a lot. I need you to be quiet for a minute." Conjure the crimson expression of a man being shushed by a peer. This elicits as much shame as any instance of acting out or sexual fantasy. In general, the conflicts that group members dread the most are the ones that may materialize at any given moment, about any topic.

In this respect, the dynamics of a group differ from those of a couple. Within a couple, familiarity loosens inhibitions, which renders process (relational) comments the norm, not the exception. With couples, the ubiquity of process comments leads to the opposite problem: excessive conflict borne of prejudiced thinking and individuals' assumptions about each other. Group members also have beliefs about one another, but fear of exclusion tends to block their expression. In couples therapy, an addict's partner might desperately ask, "What were you thinking?" when learning about an acting out or triggering event. In this context, the question carries not so much curiosity or concern, but the exasperated desire of the invested questioner. Such questions in groups are, in contrast, antidotal, as men discover that "they are not alone." Although the sentiment can feel trite when it is stated, it is nonetheless genuine. The isolation that addicts feel cannot be overstated, nor can the need to be understood. The need to be understood is reflected in all formats of therapy, but in group therapy it seems especially pronounced. Nothing stirs the thought-punctuating half-query, "If that makes sense?" quite like the gaze of an audience. The speaker who utters these words betrays an old desire to merge with another and to belong to some unit of society, and others rarely fail to respond well in these moments, for it stirs fellow-feeling to witness someone flailing with their words, not knowing if others *get them*.

Unfortunately, there are downsides to the group therapy format that must be addressed. When group members do little more than sympathize with the acting out, or someone floundering with their thoughts, a supportive but ineffective group tends to steer individuals away from their elusive selves. For example, group members may direct unconscious assumptions, or projections, at one another. As they react to a man describing his regret over a pattern of acting out and the prospect of disclosing to his wife, they might do so from the crypts of their own fears. Activating their own defenses, they turn attention away from the sharing member's thoughts and feelings to the potentially frightening responses of his wife. Someone might ask, "What did your wife say to that?" or "Did you get in trouble?" rather than deepening the member's reflection on his regret. The so-called judgment of the self is projected onto those who elicit fears of dependency, but are deflected from the lesser conscious fear of the group. Therefore, wives, girlfriends, or other committed partners (but not group members) are often cast as critics to be feared and defended against, not loved ones who merit truth and repair.

Group Therapy Versus 12-Step Participation

Group therapy requires active participation of members in ways that 12-step meetings typically do not. Group therapy calls on members to do more than share about addiction, or sex, or even recovery. At some point, the format calls on them to think about process, how they relate to peers, and how they perceive authority. Newcomers often take silent observation as their preferred stance. This recalls 12-step tradition, to offer a compromise between belonging and commitment and to diminish pressure on a participant. A newcomer may justify diffidence with humility, claiming he has less to share because he is new and therefore less knowledgeable on the topics being discussed. In our opinion this isn't the main reason that newcomers are reticent. The more salient reasons are shame, distrust, and fear. The latter does not necessarily involve fears related to competence or knowledge, but instead deeper fears: of revulsion or hate. On the one hand, a group won't work if it is comprised entirely of members waiting for others to share, take risks, and expose dark fantasies. Bionion analysts speak of mirroring group passivity, sitting quietly without providing verbal direction for a group. Such a leader challenges a group's assumptions about group leadership and provokes member responsibility. The silence appears to generate tension, which eventually topples the sense of safety that silence is initially meant to create, making the intervention paradoxical. Silence eventually leads to more interpersonal sharing. Working through their resistance (which may include blaming, or appeals directed at the therapist), members appear to learn something important about their relational beliefs: that silence amid witnesses, rather like stillness and inactivity, is even less comfortable than talking.

Group members who speak often or too much, or who ask questions drawing attention away from someone's self-experience—dubbed "blocking" by some group therapists—do not intend to support a defensive process. Their monopolistic orations or redirecting queries tend to be inadvertent, unconscious, and habitual. Some monopolists are closet distancers. They contribute much, remarking on others' sharing, being "helpful," as their peers might observe, but somehow time keeps running out before they "check in" during group sessions. Such strategies seem half-conscious, which affords them a level of deniability. This is not true of all evasive strategies. Glibness, for example, or jargon-poaching, can be a problem in groups, especially when the tactic feels deliberate. An ambivalent group member may stonewall, saying "I'm in an okay place. I've been having some issues, struggling with my addiction, trying to work on my integrity." Translation: *I slept with a prostitute*. In leaderless activities such as 12-step meetings, there is no one designated to intervene if participants avoid sharing about themselves or speak vaguely because the fellowship's principles are meant to contain the intrusions of shaming or advice-giving that are otherwise normal in society. Anonymity is given paramount weight in 12-step circles and is manifested in norms that proscribe cross-talk (commenting on members' shares). So, there is no mechanism in 12-step meetings for process comments to shape how members might speak to one another. No group figure is "othered," tolerated as different from the group, or allowed to ask questions that disturb. Therefore, if someone is making a speech, issuing platitudes about the problem of men not sharing feelings, or explaining an upbringing in which the sharing of feelings was routinely discouraged, heads may nod in acknowledgment of a familiar-sounding history, but there will be no comment like the one we might offer: that such sharing, though it may be truthful, perpetuates nonsharing by talking about phenomena in theoretical terms only.

The 12-step presumption that relapsing addicts suffer self-punishing shame is disputed by some. Skeptics may believe that being caught (not the slipping itself) is the addict's problem. This reflects a belief that shame *follows* acting out and is stirred by exposure, rather than *preceding* and therefore triggering acting out. Skeptics have good reasons to make this supposition. After all, though we often hear the phrase, "don't beat up on yourself" as a soothing gesture directed at acting out members, we rarely hear group members comment that acting out itself constitutes "beating up on yourself." (FSLA groups, perhaps?) Again, this is because groups are more inclined to support rather than confront, or just think differently.

This is not to say that honesty isn't valued. In groups, raw, self-effacing expressions that touch on but do not excessively indulge sexual detail are reveled in, welcomed as jewels that open up a process, albeit one that must be cleaned up before everyone heads home to the missus. In other words, the group is a container that must stir an optimal level of sharing, but then tidily close the lid. Also, everyone involved must believe that they belong to an optimal degree. This is tricky because outsiders, impacted partners and such, are not the only ones skeptical about criteria for group participation. Despite the compassion that addiction concepts might leverage, the idea of sex addiction is attached to a question mark. The normalcy of sex, even more than the normalcy of drug or alcohol use, dents conviction about inclusion in a "problem" group. As stated in Chapter 1, a question of addiction nags when habits become abnormal, either through frequency or because they cross value thresholds. Then the prescriptive issue is about layered exposure: can members tolerate being witnessed, and be themselves? Can they be honest?

Groups Discussing Sexual Fantasy, Sexual Abuse, and Violence

An appeal for candor is a rebranding of risk and is a group ethic aimed at anyone who otherwise links risk with self-destructive acts. Morals, judgment, and ethics are concepts that are often confused, perhaps reflecting weariness of morality as an institutionalized oppressor, but not with the choice to do right in some less prescribed manner. In our groups, we canvas opinion in hopes of making the implicit explicit. According to one assumption, morals are about sex. According to another, ethics are more about money, or generalized notions of fairness, like equality. So, does the use of prostitutes blend morality and ethics, for example? Within a group with a therapeutic purpose, members typically agree that everyone should feel equal and that privacy ought to be protected. These standards rarely seem oppressive. So-called judgment is a gray area of ethics. Rules are measured. It's important to be honest to and about others, but don't shame anyone. And when choosing to "call someone out," be selective.

Regarding the ethics of sex and aggression beyond the confines of group, it's rare to hear members admit to harassing women to have sex, or otherwise perpetrating anything like a nonconsensual sex act. Given the rates of sexual abuse victimization reported by women, and the rates of sexual abuse survival increasingly being reported by men, something is amiss. Where are the corresponding perpetrators, and what are their stories? Of course, we know why undiscovered perpetrators don't raise their hands in anything resembling a public setting, but amid the pregnant silence and stonewalling, *I've-got-nothing-to-say* expressions, a group leader can wait for glimpses of members' split-off (denied, "not me") aggressions.

> Once, a man I thought less likely to engage in such behavior made a confession: "I remember times I pressured women to have sex with me." He went on to detail the events and the shame he felt as he reflected on this. As he did so, I scanned the room, looking to see who might respond, ask questions, or join in the spirit of disclosure. One or two guys jumped in, sharing the shame with that brave first member, copping to all the copped feels and other such misconduct. Ironically, I think it was a relative lack of shame that loosened their tongues. The quietest members in the room stirred the most curiosity in me. I thought that those with the least to say had the darkest secrets.

Sexual violence may seem tangential to sexual addiction, especially as sex offending or gender-based violence is, for the most part, not conflated with sex addiction within the field of treatment. However, like the topics of prostitution, misogyny, or objectification, the subject of sexual abuse does seem to intersect with sex addiction to some degree. However, the matter of sex and violence feels like one of those barely begun, blunted conversations between men and women. Take, for example, a common scenario of sexual assault:

> A man and a woman flirt with each other, go on a date, and finish the evening in a private room. Intimacy escalates, but the woman decides late against sex and objects. Too late, or so thinks the man who doesn't stop and . . . basically, a rape follows.

Society seems divided on this type of scenario. Many (both men and women) blame the woman for allowing the escalation of sex, leading to violence. Another, more vocal (at least recently) constituency protests that this point of view falsely blames the victim, and more plainly faults the man for not containing his impulses. A neutral third voice blandly observes that if intimate partners speak more clearly, and don't get lost in the haze of flirtation, they might avert disaster.

This latter view seems correct, yet it says everything and nothing. As for the lens of public opinion, history seems checkered. Today, a commonly heard narrative blames toxic masculinity, a brand of male-inflected narcissism, for escalations of sexual violence. The idea that a man who is rejected is prone to violence substitutes for the view that would fault the woman for causing violence because she *changes her mind*. The men we speak to on this subject tend to emphasize or at least introduce this latter point, whether they've been accused of assault or not. They don't so much own the rejection as observe the manipulative nature of women, claiming a dynamic event with blame at its center. Conscious and unconscious forces congeal and clash, with feelings crushed and replaced by defenses. A primitive self-representation of being "bad" or "unworthy" (introjection) dovetails with an anger-filled projection of a "bad" other who not only rejects but has devised the conditions leading to the rejection. The rape becomes an act of power triggered by another act of power that the perpetrator assigns to the victim. This interpretation may spare victims from blame in some quarters, but it does not entirely exonerate. For those Ferenczi (1930, 1933) once described, it does not exonerate. Exoneration, even if accepted by an assault victim, does not extinguish feelings of shame for having enjoyed the initial mischief—the flirting with a disaster that became a disaster.

Try having that conversation in a coed group. Talk about deep breaths and *I've-got-nothing-to-say* expressions.

> Only two or three people speak, issuing platitudes or strident comments that no one dares to contest. Everyone else is too careful, wondering if the group is safe or its leaders sufficiently robust to tease out true thoughts versus driving an echo chamber. Splitting is internal and muted, only revealing itself in more private quarters. A man chuckles and observes with studied conviction, "I'm not putting my head in that noose." A woman notices reticence in the male group members. Inferring resistance to what she deems a given, she bitterly intones, "They don't want to hear it."

It's hard to imagine a coed group that would navigate these divides in a brave yet containable fashion. Men's and women's conversations seem to retreat to their separate chambers to nurse and echo their long-standing and somewhat analogous grievances. For this and other reasons, sex addiction therapy groups generally segregate by sex. Less threateningly, but also stereotypically, women find men's habit of suggesting emotional commitment and then withdrawing to be offensive, and perhaps punishable if the world was governed by Jane Austen fans. Men find women's habit of suggesting sex and then withdrawing from sex to be frustrating; it elicits dark contemplations that defy traditional norms, and conjures a silent, amoral query that preludes violence: what is the point of a God-given physical advantage?

A Sex Addiction Superego: Group Conscience and Purpose

A psychodynamic sex addiction therapy group has a practical function similar to any behavior-monitoring support group, but also a more abstracted role. As a stand-in for the community eye, a cohesive group is a modified superego: an observant conscience comprised of similarly afflicted peers, not an external set of judges acting with moral severity. The intent is that a group represents the community and that individual members will integrate aspirational values and embrace the secure attachment rather than a dopamine rush adhered to fantasies of perfection or frozen youth. If bonding occurs, it results from a felt experience with others. Members may begin a therapeutic process thinking that stressors are consciously accessible. "Well, let's see, everything's been okay this week," a group member might say, thinking of external events. He might learn only later that his addictive pattern reacts to an unconscious complex of entitlement and displacement. A front of entitlement conceals an ashamed, disentitled self, and relational needs are displaced onto sexual compulsion. A successful, recovering member might not be able to explain why he has achieved a pleasing streak of sober, nonacting-out time. Despite employing tools that enable his sober, outer circle activities (such as journaling, making phone calls, or consistently seizing time in group), he may be no more observant of being healthy than he was of the dissociative spells that enabled his acting out behaviors. We think this paradox lies at the core of a treatment's efficacy, which may be quietly and unceremoniously observed. A "successful" outcome—whether gauged at 90 days, 6 months, or 5 years—is borne of action, but also of mystery.

Wary of others, individuals in groups may speak less of sex than they might in private, one-on-one sessions. As in the case of Tony, described in Chapter 3, the most unbearable acts to speak of may be displaced by less offensive, more commonplace behaviors, like masturbation to porn. Alternatively, members may celebrate others' good news as evidence of hope, like the resumption of sex following a moratorium. Such announcements are usually greeted with triumphant smiles and pumping fists. Again, this is all about fitting in, not standing out, as the latter action leads away from the pack, which further leads to ostracism, the unconscious fear of death. Consider the following risky disclosure:

> A group member who frequented massage parlors talked about "happy endings" (slang for reaching climax through manual stimulation). He spoke of receiving this service while suckling on the worker's nipples, and about the regressive elements of his fantasy. No talking. That was the secret ingredient, he realized: the mute exchange between himself and a woman, which he'd been searching for but not once explicitly requested. The pedigree of this behavior was infantile, altering a previous belief that philandering men, like his father, were his models. But this group member wasn't a womanizer, so he revised his conception of himself. Sex was a return to the earliest form of pleasure he could imagine, not a wish to silence women. His tone was matter-of-fact as he was half-lost in his reverie. His peers looked stunned; their jaws tightened like they were straining to keep their mouths from dropping open. *Who is this Dr. Strangelove?* What could they actually say? Could the man avoid that kind of behavior in the future? No. What were the stressors, or "triggers" that may have led to that acting out behavior? Also not right. I could see the wheels turning, the mental circuits short-circuiting. Had that man really invoked the ancient taboo,[2] and

---

2. The taboo again refers to *Oedipus Rex*. From this myth, most interpretations observe the fantasies of an infantilized male, who makes active a once passive sexuality. In a feminine analogy to the Oedipal complex, women are said to manifest trauma via somatic disturbances. Kristeva (1974) rebuked psychoanalysis for its exclusive focus on the maternal/child bond, which ignores a mother's psychic eroticism, reduces women to passive roles, and may obscure eroticism more readily assigned to the genital sexuality of men. Prior to the Oedipal crisis, the root

> could anyone go the last mile of this conversation and name it? Were they supposed to do something, or was I? I interpreted the event as written, but beyond that, I offered no prescription.

Like Bader (2009), we think that eliciting fantasies like the one described above is close to the raison d'etre of psychodynamic therapy, including sex addiction group therapy. This may surprise those who believe that the real mandates of a responsible program or clinician are to provide concrete "tools" for recovery, contain acting out, or facilitate disclosure to non-acting out partners—basically, to arrest the behavior. The rationale for our approach is as follows:

- Discussing fantasies, or "triggers," may—or may not—cause physical acting out. Not discussing them might have the same effect.
- Therapy participants of all types (including self-identified addicts) resist being directed, especially over time.
- Contrary to pockets of professional opinion, not all sex addicts exhibit risks to their own medical, legal, or occupational functioning.
- As it is commonly described, sex addiction does not meet medical necessity criteria.

In chemical dependency programs, it is common for counselors to intervene (aka censor) if and when patients begin stories that contain details of a using episode, including the use of slang or references to particular drugs or drug ephemera. Corey (2008) suggested that a censoring ethic should exist in any group process if the group's purpose is to be achieved. If such shares seem comic or "glorifying," someone in the group will likely protest, suggesting that they trigger cravings, and generally stir desire that may lead to relapse, which presumes that treatment participants have a baseline motivation to abstain. These types of shares, sometimes

---

of man's infantile sexuality may lie in an "original intimate unity," according to Loewald (1979). Alternatively, it may lie in the gratification afforded him in early childhood when the source of nourishment was also a source of sexual pleasure; when relinquished, according to Klein (1935, 1940), that [nourishment? pleasure?] leaves an infant in the care of a frightening figure. Is sex addiction a cycle of anger, guilt, hate, and indulgence that is later reenacted? And has the aroused "memory" become more exciting than the repressed original event?

dubbed "war stories," are largely discouraged for the sake of protecting abstinence.

We don't think the same rationale applies to the treatment of sex addicts, as the goals (abstinence? monogamy?) are more ambiguous. While we agree that using names of hook-up websites ought to be discouraged, and that contact details of a massage establishment should not be shared casually or flippantly, the acting out behavior or fantasy-related shares of sex addicts should rarely be censored. Why? Shame is likely to be induced in the group to an optimal degree (the value of which is implied by the disparagement "shameless"), but talking about drinking or drugging among a group of alcoholics or drug addicts doesn't elicit the same degree of embarrassment as sharing the details of sexual acting out. It's not even in the same league. We believe that there is conscious and unconscious aggression in sex addicts' repertoires, but unlike the drug user who revels in being high around an authority figure, they do not brag in groups about acting out right under the noses of their bosses or partners. Neither do they sit around in groups arguing for the legalization of prostitution the way that some proselytize their drugs of choice. Invariably, would-be sex addicts enter treatment nervously, wary of the judgments of men as well as women. Affair-seekers may have it a little easier, as their pattern of acting out is at least syntonic with the ego of mainstream masculine culture. Although porn and prostitute-users are enfolded into the media's "toxic masculinity" polemic, we find them to be passive, shuffling into our offices without bravado and often looking like they're picturing others picturing them doing something unmentionable.

We also don't buy the notion that adult sex addicts get their ideas from listening to other sex addicts share their fantasies. For those who enter our offices and participate in our groups, that ship has sailed. Thoughts of acting out may be stirred by listening to another's fantasies or reviewing their own in individual therapy, but that downside is outweighed by the benefits of talking about those fantasies, unearthing them from their shameful lairs and studying them (versus getting lost in them) in the presence of others. The rationale is partly the same as the justification for the cognitive exploration of thoughts that generate anxiety and depression: to examine possible distortions and to understand meaning. Providers who treat survivors of abuse, or the most compulsive or psychotic of dependents, may disagree, of course. Among our peers we perceive a similar conservatism. Many discourage the sharing of fantasy, half-believing that thought equals action (psychic equivalence), or that fantasy renders sex addicts vulnerable to relapse or to a spiral into destructive paths (jails, institutions, or death, plus collateral damage). Sex addiction, self-harm, and violence intertwine—or intersect—psychologically, and at times behaviorally. For some, sex addiction proceeds like domino theory: it is like a once-upon-a-time Vietnamese Front, with the addict's self-destruction, plus the mass rape of women and children on the horizon. Thankfully, the diagnostic governances of our profession have not deemed sex addiction so dangerous or destructive from a medical, legal, or social standpoint that it compels detoxifying, repressive measures for most treatment subjects.

CASE ILLUSTRATION: A WOMEN'S GROUP EXPERIENCE

The misandrist women referenced in Chapters 2 and 4 don't represent most of the women we've observed in sex addiction treatment. That particular societal faction doesn't last long in the process for a very simple reason: they lack the open-mindedness that would render them viable candidates for therapy.

> I had the opportunity to lead a women's group for an interim spell under similar circumstances as that previous experience (lack of a female group leader). I sat with women who had been earnestly addressing the impact of sex addiction for several years. The mix of women in this group was diverse, not culturally or ethnically, but in terms of attitudes. The group included passive deniers, those who were angry yet wise, the bewildered, and the ashamed. I gleaned that several difficult personalities had passed through the group's turnstiles over the years, adopting the victim/survivor narratives and masking their characters (or not). In some cases, their characters were as disordered as those of their male-partner counterparts in the program. In holding the group leader spot until a suitable female therapist came along, I was braced for a delicate, poignant, and possibly dangerous encounter.

The sex addict partner group's superego is different from that of men's groups: it challenges participants to divest emotionally from their partners and their continued acting out. It also promotes independence; dissolution of rivalry between women;[3] a stoic surrender of the romanticist and religiously influenced ideals that sexual acting out has violated; and perseverance in the face of disappointment. Among the things these women never wanted to do was join a support group and listen to other women share stories that either mirrored their own or made them wonder what they were missing. They never wanted to tell their husbands or boyfriends about other women's horror stories and then hear defensive replies like, "Well, I'm not as bad as those guys." Some of the women we've met in this context want repair in relationships. Others are grieving, as their partnerships have already dissolved.

> Some in this particular group still wanted their men to be "into them," as they put it, seemingly half-aware of their desire for emotional and sexual penetration. During a discussion of honesty, I maximized my substitute role, challenging them to say what they were ready to hear from the men, or what they'd risk listening to if they could have past conversations all over again. In particular, I wanted to know if they felt ready to hear about sexual fantasies, their partners' behavioral slips (such as those double-takes on the "hot" women in the office), the "intriguing" pictures they saw online, or the flirtatious exchanges in which they may have indulged. Would they risk hearing what men privately wanted (whether they'd gratify their wishes or not)? And what if these thoughts and behaviors were volunteered rather than divulged reluctantly after a series of hard questions or an investigative discovery? The women in the circle nodded agreeably, saying they'd find it refreshing, a relief even, if the men in their lives would ever—or had ever, just once, felt comfortable enough (or trusting enough, I suggested)—to share with them the thoughts and feelings

3. Another example of the modern superego: at a SASH conference in 2015, I heard a presenter deliver psychoeducational marching orders for an audience of sex addiction specialists. The speaker pronounced that women should "blame the cheaters" not the "other women." The speaker went on to say that the tendency to blame women for infidelity reflects competition between women for partners, which in turn reflects the oppressive influence of men, and that progressive, civilized thought should therefore alter this aged dynamic. Competition between men for female sexual partners was also referenced in this talk, but in that context the presenter was concerned with the conspiratorial desire to control or conquer women, not the damage done to bonds between men.

> about which they felt so much shame and guilt. The women declared that they would welcome such an exchange.
>
> All except one woman, I discovered. I had seen it coming. No group is entirely cohesive (uniform in level of understanding or capacity). Speaking nervously, the dissenter asked about the implications of my premise that the men in question had acted out in ways that were either unknown or (worse) continuing. "My husband says he's focused on extinguishing these thoughts. I'm not saying he's cured but. . . ." She looked around the room, suddenly aware that she was sharing a foolish thought, that her husband's addiction was a past tense phenomenon. It was no doubt a comforting thought, but it was not in keeping either with the group superego or the recovery ethos, which asserts that addiction is a lifelong problem and is not extinguishable in the way this woman appeared to need. Some of the other women in the room looked away, embarrassed and not knowing what to say. They'd been here before. The group discussion trailed off and the isolated woman expressed. "I don't understand," she said, teetering on emotional collapse. The group norm shifted to caretaking, focusing on empathy for a partner's understandable fears, mostly delivered with platitudes. She later blamed my gratuitous provocations for making her feel unsafe.

One of the downsides of the group process is that it can't promise to carry everyone at the same pace. Not everyone integrates the same principles and applies them equally. Inevitably, someone will learn or think of something that penetrates a fog.

Although a group's principal charter is safety, we actually think that therapy is meant to stir optimal discomfort, with an estimated threshold of safety. The degree of success varies, depending on individual capacities and defenses. The defense of splitting (keeping separate that which will do harm) is reinforced by a norm in which men primarily work with men, and women keep to themselves with female-only facilitators. Because men and women will harm one another, they must be kept separate. The interim presence of a male therapist in that women's group may have felt like an intrusion to some or, at best, a diplomatic mission from an adversarial, foreign emissary. That such leadership yielded a casualty may have reinforced some group members' beliefs that male voices didn't belong. Others may have seen it as the kind of medicine the group needed. And other views may have fallen somewhere in between. As suggested earlier in the chapter and in Ley (2012), the demographics of our profession make it more likely that women will facilitate men's groups rather than the converse arrangement. This echoes an observation by Markale (1972): a surrender to the feminine in which the heterosexual masculine ethic—impenetrability—is called for and challenged. From an analytic perspective, challenging psychological defenses and facilitating intimacy in the company of men is a castrating action, leading to a feminine identification. While the perceived purpose of men's groups is to yield a later healing between man and woman, the wraparound agenda of the group stirs another taboo that bears support: penetration from and surrender to fellow men.

Conflict Resolution and Groups as Microcosms of Commitment

The men that stick around in groups and bond with other members, whether a core clique or a revolving door of newcomers, tend to develop subtly elite self-images over time, akin to what Freud (1930) called the "narcissism of minor differences" to describe phenomena such as nationalism and tribal pride. These men listen to their wives and girlfriends complain about their corresponding support groups as they relate "horror" stories of other men's serial betrayals and inveterate relapsing. Veteran group members evince sympathy inflected with distance—what some call "othering." Those addicts who keep going *out there*, hurting themselves and their loved ones, are the misbegotten and are deserving of compassion, but they are different from men who are in treatment, working on themselves. These men constitute a different class of addict. This separation notwithstanding, what most group members would admit having in common with their lost group members is a tendency toward that very same habit: distancing. What hurts groups most is the same thing that happens in the lives of sex addicts and their loved ones: addicts are often absent, and may leave precipitously, usually without explaining why. Absenteeism in groups is stressful and often stirs anxiety in group members. However, feelings of abandonment are typically denied, instead transformed into "concern" for the missing group member, that guy who is out in the wilderness, presumably sliding back into his addiction, lost in shame and spiraling out of control. It's like an echo of the soldier's code: concern for a lost comrade. This concern is genuine, but it obscures group members' other anxieties: about getting lost themselves, and—less consciously, perhaps—about feelings of closeness with other men.

When the undercurrent of closeness is suggested in men's groups, a leader may be met with furrowed-brow stares and nonplussed silence. Members don't disagree with the idea so much as act as if it hadn't been stated. Group members might simply reiterate their concern for the person who is absent and wonder about those innumerable cues in the environment that may trigger slips (such as beautiful women in the street or ads on the internet), but not so much about what is happening when someone is . . . *gone*. If something doesn't compute, it's easier to ignore it. If certain feelings are intolerable, it's best to swat them away before they even register. We don't insist that this is the case. Insisting that feelings denied are necessarily present on an unconscious level is another circular argument. As therapists, it's enough to float the idea of intimacy fear, observe the stolid misunderstanding, listen to the denials, and watch a few Adam's apples move and some shoulders shrug. We can't prove that people are vulnerable to rejection, loneliness, or hate. Some might admit these feelings theoretically, knowing or feeling what is true, but still erect their defenses, excusing the absent and focusing on the other's needs instead of their own. Abandonment secretly touches on a deeper wound: a feeling that group members are unimportant and not worth showing up for.

What a group leader should ask for, typically during a pre-group orientation, is an understanding of group commitment. This means asking prospective group members to attend group for a minimum period, such as 90 days (or preferably longer in the case of weekly groups), and to give a month's notice if leaving for whatever reason. This introduces another ethic—*don't abandon*. This commitment has little if anything to do with principles of resilience, such as the idea of "giving therapy a chance" because "change doesn't happen overnight." Minimum attendance and giving space for termination has more to do with the highly personal information that is exchanged in groups. Members are being asked to share not just with a paid professional, but with a vulnerable group of peers with implicit needs, such as the need to know whether it's worth bonding with someone who may or may not stick around. Unfortunately, although newcomers tend to nod agreeably during orientation, there's no legislating for forgetting. Shamefaced sex addicts might agree to just about anything at the outset of treatment, just to deescalate the distress of this period. That's why group commitments need to be reiterated at regular intervals. Still, shockingly (or not), group members do indeed "ghost" from groups, conflict, and themselves. The rationales, if thought about, may vary from "I don't remember that policy" to "Sorry, I got a new job and I just don't have any time." But the problem is profound. Of course, not showing up, not returning calls, and disappearing are not unique to sex addict groups. Busy people make daily decisions about what and who are important, and battles are chosen. Sometimes decisions are made in the name of emotional safety, reflecting a context-traversing attachment style. Analogies include the workplace that unceremoniously escorts laid-off employees from an office and the impersonal nature of online dating. Distancing is downloaded into culture and is usually framed as a matter of security. The truth is that managing conflicts, staying close, and attending to interpersonal needs, regardless of context (personal, occupational, historical, and present-day), just doesn't seem to matter enough.

CASE ILLUSTRATION: ERIC, STU, AND A FEW SUPPORTIVE MEN

Although they had been in group together for years, Eric and Stu did not seem to like each other. For the most part, they were cordial but aloof, with sparse feedback for each other's relational needs or sources of shame. I thought of them as sparks and gasoline, ever ready to ignite. As their group leader, I'd helped them coexist, occasionally pointing out their differences. I had observed neutrally Stu's hot temper and his tendency toward sudden escalation, fight, and then repair. Eric seemed more reserved and prone to quips that sometimes landed awkwardly but didn't appear to offend. Well, they offended Stu. More than anyone realized, including myself, Eric's sideways comments, incongruent smiles, laughter, and odd gestures drove Stu crazy. One day, Stu was distressed in group, expressing fear that his wife would leave him following her discovery of his latest behavioral slip. As Stu was prone to venting angrily about his wife, some in the group may have been surprised to see him anxious about losing her. Eric suggested as much, asking, "Why does it matter?" and adding that he was bored by the discussion. His voice seemed correspondingly flat and uninterested, and his garden gnome smile seemed opaque. As Eric spoke, I observed Stu's facial twitches and an emergent shaking in his knees. Fleetingly, I thought of a musical analogy: a drum-roll heralding an impending thunderclap. It occurred to me that I should comment on Eric's demeanor, observe its contrast with Stu and the rest of the group, and perhaps avert a group-rupturing disaster.

Too late. Seconds later, Stu was spitting feathers, bellowing rage at his peer's insensitivity and threatening to leave the group and never return. As he stormed toward the exit I stood up and—not quite matching his volume—appealed to him to stay in the room and get support from the group (not excluding Stu, but not specifying him for the moment). At that moment, most of the group's members did not seem prepared to support anyone. They all looked concussed, not knowing what to do or say. They also wanted to leave. The least uncomfortable-looking person was Eric, who continued to sit benignly, looking like a host organism of hate, not its conscious exponent. In all respects, it seemed as if feeling would neither go into nor flow out from him. By this point, Stu was still frothing, positioned at the door, looking past me and over my shoulder, like a mad dog staring down its prey. Wisely or not, I captured his attention, convinced him to stay in the room, calm down, and talk through what had just happened. I'd played this referee/lion-tamer role numerous times earlier in my career when working in group homes, corralling impulsive teens to sit with and tolerate one another. I drew on that memory and experience, thinking it would be a success if I could just contain the heat and keep it in the room until it ebbed. Some group members may have preferred that Stu leave to reduce the tension. It seemed that the group looked to me to create peace, save the group from collapse and rescue everyone individually from their respective traumas. That didn't happen. By the end of that group session, Eric's apology to Stu soothed nerves, but it did not yield understanding. That task was left to the détente that followed. However, détente doesn't promise resolution. Instead, it is merely a ceasefire between battles.

Almost everyone involved kept attending. Half aware of its needs, the group seemed to want this mini-community to survive. Although it might tolerate individuals leaving or—to a lesser degree—individuals being expelled if they were disruptive or otherwise unacceptable, the group needed its core purpose to continue. Eric and Stu continued to coexist, occasionally giving each other supportive feedback and even managing to enjoy each other's humor at times. I remained uneasy about their participation, however, especially because their subsequent process continued without yielding insight about their previous conflict. My uneasiness heightened as Stu began sharing childhood memories that were being unearthed in his concurrent individual therapy. Around age 11, he had been molested by an older boy, a child of one of his parents' friends in whose company Stu had been regularly placed while the adults socialized separately. In his shares, Stu was not explicit about the molestation, yet he increasingly cited this multi-incident episode as the root cause of his later addictive habits. It was unusual, but not unheard of, for group members to report episodes of abuse during rather than in advance of group participation. For the most part, the group seemed supportive of Stu as he made these disclosures, but they were neutral about the links between abuse and addiction. Spying Eric in my peripheral vision, I gleaned from his reticence that he was skeptical.

Eric was the only member of the group with a sex offending history. A self-proclaimed nudist, he'd been arrested more than once for indecent exposure and had been warned by police for publicly wearing scant clothing that partly exposed his genitals. In treatment, Eric readily admitted his exhibitionist nature but denied intending any harm to others. Despite this presentation, other group members appeared to accept Eric. He was an amiable man who was generally indulged, not rejected, when he made offhand remarks. Though his behavioral profile may have been different, his nondirect contact offenses did not cross others' threshold of repugnance. While his interpersonal style resonated with other members' avoidant defenses, he bonded with them and they, in turn, seemed able to tolerate his objectionable history.

His participation walked a fine line, as group members who accept the label of sex addict generally bristle at the label perpetrator. In addition, they tend to resist association with peers who have been designated as sex offenders by law. In contemporary society, they are surely the last faction that we are allowed to hate and talk about hating. Figuratively, they are our modern lepers, deemed unworthy of treatment intervention or psychotherapy.

> Well beyond his original mandate and without arrests or police warnings in years, Eric was no longer a nuisance in public areas, it seemed, but his offhand manner and perpetrator's image was a risk to the group, or at least to Stu, I thought. At times, I found pretexts for observing the undercurrent, wondering aloud if Eric's seeming identification with accused figures in media would clash with Stu's growing sympathy for victims. Whether those pretexts were visceral enough as triggers, it seemed that denial ran deep, as neither group member seemed moved by my suggestion until one group session when the topic of discussion was a media focus on sexual abuse victims. In broaching the subject, Stu revealed his bias, bemoaning the abuse aimed at individuals who were making accusations about decades' old events. Predictably, Eric made a twofold rebuttal, complaining that statute of limitations, as a principle, ought to be observed. He then insinuated that accusers would seek legal settlements and were therefore motivated by profit. This latter suggestion triggered Stu. Within moments he was hurling insults and shouting over my attempts to assuage him. Above all, it seemed to be Eric's offhand, frivolous manner that had disturbed Stu, though throughout this episode I continued to believe that Eric's identification was a contributing factor.

How do you stop a tsunami or a wildfire? You develop early warning systems, build levees, or tell people to evacuate before a crisis hits. You build walls, separate sparks from gasoline, and reconcile truth and lies later, when conditions seem safer. After all, there is a reason for splitting, taught the likes of Klein (1935, 1946) and Bion (1959, 1961b).

> Intuitively, I let Stu bail from the room after this latest outburst, thinking that he should leave the group temporarily. It certainly didn't seem like the time to don my old group home persona and perform an "okay guys, let's chill out and shake hands" kind of moment. This time I *knew* the divide was deeper. The latest spark had perhaps ignited the spilt pool of gasoline. "That was unfortunate," I muttered with massive

understatement. What was my unconscious process? Would I under-react, resonating with the passive elements in the room? Or would I pick up the baton left by Stu and modify his position by criticizing Eric for his provocative comments firmly but with a detached air? My initial soft-spoken response betrayed my preference. I was insinuating quiet as the way forward and implicitly taking sides.

Over the ensuing weeks, the group processed the conflict. Adversaries Stu and Eric took part in alternate group sessions. I had split the group with Kleinian suppositions in mind. I was not asserting good or bad in a judicious sense, but with a sense of what arrangement might leverage sharing. Conflict is painful and dangerous. Underlying the discussion was a recognition that avoidance had served as an accomplice to nearly everyone's addiction. Every group member could cite examples of acting out that had replaced the stress of dealing with people, but they thought that treatment, therapy, or group was a refuge from such triggers. Someone, whether me as leader or Eric and Stu as antagonists, had broken the tacit agreement of the group. The other members seemed both anxious and angry, not liking this *live* test of their defenses. Who was to blame? Who should evacuate or be eliminated? Predictably enough, Stu made his position clear: he would no longer participate in group if Eric remained a member. He had no problem with anyone else; Eric was the problem. The following week, Eric suggested that he was available for reconciliation and bore no ill-will toward Stu. Since he'd previously established his "I don't intend harm" mode across contexts (which hadn't protected him legally), his position was also unsurprising. The other members of the group didn't quite buy his stance. Challenging Eric about why he'd debated Stu, they observed an aggressive streak in him. They felt that he should have been more "sensitive" to Stu's history. Even if he disagreed with Stu's hotly expressed opinions, as they sometimes did, Eric didn't have to argue with him. The group's position, its view of a collective self, was that group members vent about stuff and we don't have to agree with them. We just have to listen.

"My aggressive streak?" Eric asked incredulously. His affect became heightened. He didn't reach Stu's level of intensity, but there was life in Eric. His laughter took on a more obviously derisive quality, which the group may have observed but did not comment on directly. I did. Entering the process, I said that he seemed angry and that his tone seemed mocking. I added that this impression was especially apparent in this moment, but it was a regular occurrence. Wide-eyed, shrugging like a child who has sat in the back of class his whole life, Eric said, "Maybe I'm a shitty group member." A moment of silence followed. Intuiting the manipulative nature of his gesture, no one moved to dispel or confirm Eric's supposition. He seemed embarrassed that the cat—his aggression—had been let out of the bag. His brief outburst stood in ironic contrast to Stu's quietude in a previous session that Eric did not attend. During that process, Stu had been poised yet contrite with respect to the group as a whole. Partly via my prompting, he'd given thought to his role in the group over time. He was regretful that his diatribes and his temper had intimidated other group members, possibly deterring some from being candid with him. Though Stu was resolute in his stance about Eric, he did not implore the group to see things his way. Insisting that he respected everyone present, he agreed to take a hiatus from the group and accept the result of the process.

In the weeks that followed, pressure mounted on Eric. Though no one asked him to leave, the group's bias toward Stu was apparent and I think Eric felt the group's disapproval. I kept in contact with Stu, asking him to reconsider a return, but he was adamantly opposed. He declared that he'd stayed once before because of my influence—not again. As a compromise, I offered to facilitate a meeting between Eric and Stu, pointing out that Eric was once again contrite and seemingly open to learning about his less obviously aggressive habits. "Well, that idea is even worse," Stu replied, now thinking I was crazy. I was so determined (desperate?) to stop splitting from prevailing that I was willing to try anything to get the spark and the gasoline together. However, it seemed equally important to get the voyeurs off the sidelines and keep the group involved. This impending rupture somehow felt more painful and had been more discouraging than any couple's split that I'd witnessed.

There was one gratifying aspect of this group divorce, however. The other members were willing to engage in the process, look past temper tantrums, and perceive that there was aggression on all sides. One style of aggression was not necessarily preferable to another. They saw Eric and Stu in themselves and shared my disappointment about group dissolution. Eric seemed to shrink from the group process, speaking less and less. His isolation included mute or forced responses to others' shares. A month or so after that last incident with Stu, he matter-of-factly announced that he'd be leaving the group permanently and immediately.

The case of Eric and Stu has parallels with the case of Rick and Anne in Chapters 1 and 4. Like Rick, Eric is the avoidantly attached figure, less aware of his traumatic background, but acting on it as he dissociates intimacy needs, escaping into misty fantasy. Like Anne, Stu is the ambivalently attached figure, pining for closeness and honesty, but wary of danger and prone to more demonstrative retreats.

Despite everything that had gone wrong, I was pleased that my group had avoided dichotomies, those binary lines in the sand that are so easy to draw. In a sense, they had evolved as an addiction support group. Their thoughts had been aroused but also obscured, first by a litany of behaviors, then by a limited way of thinking, and, finally, by lasting uncertainties. In facing their crisis, the group moved beyond jargon and rules, first losing and then finding itself in uncharted territory. Eric's exhibitionism was likely an acting out of all he kept hidden but longed to display. In group, he was seen more fully by those prone to gazing at women, but for a change they tried looking inside with one another.

As Eric announced that he was leaving, everyone nodded assent. No one mentioned that he was breaking the rule about four weeks' notice, because his timing seemed about right. It was an imperfect end: the adversaries separated, taking their parts in the conflict with them and leaving behind an illusion of calm and harmony. The defeated party was gone and the agitator had been called out, but nobody *won*. As the leader of the group (the supposed outsider within), I was the only person in the room to really question Eric's purpose for leaving. It could be argued that Stu had left because he could no longer tolerate feeling gaslighted by a fellow group member. But Eric? Perhaps he couldn't tolerate the group's verdict that he was culpable in Stu's exit. "I think it's best," Eric concluded with an obligatory shrug. He seemed impervious to interpretation. He had made up his mind that leaving was a solution to the problem. Splitting also means not tolerating loss, or not living wholly, with natural guilt for the impact of one's desires. Interdependence of group members can be denied or individuals can be expelled or "let go," as long as group cohesion and group purpose prevail. This group had been asked to think not just about patterns of problem sexual behavior, but also about love and hate, forgiveness, envy, judgment, prejudices, trauma, groupthink, and group and world involvement. There was no happy ending. In leaving, Eric disavowed responsibility, and therefore remorse, but did he feel guilty, ashamed, unsafe, or angry? Who knows? Perhaps he was satisfied, and if his absence was a sacrifice, then it may have seemed to all an echo of familiar symbols, like comradely gestures amid war.

CHAPTER 6

Collaborative Approaches: Working With a Treatment Team

Ali Warren writes, "Shut up alone with . . . my own habits, I can get caught in a hall of looping self-doubt. But when I'm attending to another in . . . collaboration, I'm brought open to possibility, to new bonds and intimacies." Sometimes we get lost with a case and don't even realize we are lost until we speak to another member of the treatment team. Or we feel stuck until we pick up the phone to a colleague. Warren goes on to say, "Collaboration is for me a way of being permeable and open to change. It is a powerfully direct way to engage other practices of reading, listening, and thinking. If I'm being bold, I might even say that collaboration is one way to expand the boundaries and limitations of subjectivity." (Ali Warren, www.PoetryFoundation.org)

I believe our professional growth as clinicians depends upon our openness to collaboration. We may feel we are quite competent with "easy" cases, but with complex cases it's even more important to get feedback from other clinicians. In some respects, it takes a village to provide successful treatment for the identified sex addict and his family. Here are some examples of what that "village" might look like:

- The sex addict may need individual therapy to explore the intimate complexities surrounding his acting out. This seems obvious but some opt out of individual psychotherapy for group therapy exclusively.
- He may need a psychiatrist to prescribe medication for comorbid anxiety or mood disorders.

- He may benefit from group therapy to hear information from other identified sex addicts that he would never hear in individual therapy. The feedback from or confrontations with group members may be much more effective than any comments made by his individual therapist. This is highly recommended by these authors.
- His partner will likely need individual therapy to deal with the raw feelings that often arise after discovery.
- His partner may also benefit from group therapy so she can speak with other partners who have been betrayed.
- His partner may also require consultation with a psychiatrist for medication, evaluation, and monitoring.

When providers coordinate their care and collaborate, treatment usually goes well. But how can patient confidentiality be maintained with so much collaboration? Confidentiality is the bedrock of psychotherapy. The patient will be willing to share his most private secrets only if he fully trusts the therapist to protect his privacy. That being said, we routinely break confidentiality (of course, always with the consent of the patient) to consult with other members of the treatment team. If done judiciously, collaboration can further treatment goals and patient success. If done carelessly, it can stall or even explode treatment. The best way to collaborate with other team members is to have a consent for release of information agreement that lays out in detail the specific information that will be shared and the conditions under which sharing will occur. For example, it should describe how and when a therapist will speak with the spouse's therapist, a group therapist, or a couples therapist on a patient's team.

The plan for collaboration must be strategic to facilitate both individual and adjunct therapies. Butler (2010) surveyed therapists about the relational impact of disclosure versus secrets and found that "relational therapists' clinical judgment is that healing and attachment security are best promoted by disclosure, and that therapists support facilitated disclosure of infidelity in a context of informed, voluntary consent."

The agreement for sharing between the individual therapist and the couples' therapist may be different than the one between the individual and spouse's therapists. For example, both individual therapists may choose to speak in a limited way to the couples therapist about issues that involve the relationship and to facilitate goal setting for couples treatment. In this context it should be understood by all parties that slips or sexual acting out will not be specifically reported. Since the betrayed partner assumes a risk of contracting an STD from the partner's acting out, he/she may want to agree to only safe sexual practices between them. On the other hand, the individual therapists in collaboration with their clients may determine that no sharing between them and the couples therapist would be preferred to provide a sense of emotional safety and to facilitate the therapeutic relationship. A one-size-fits-all approach is less effective than an individualized plan, but the latter can be difficult to accomplish. When treatment takes place in a clinic setting, where staff meet regularly to discuss their patients, it's easy for staff to forget the individual terms of the agreements for each patient. With the best of intentions, they may slip into discussions that violate confidentiality agreements. For this reason, and to keep it simple, therapists generally use standard release of information forms. Patients are required to sign these forms, along with a stack of others, at the outset of treatment.

As an example, a patient, Jerry, indicates he signed all of these forms at a time of severe stress, along with pressure from his spouse to "go into treatment or I'm calling the divorce attorney." He was surprised when he had a slip three months later and discovered, much to his dismay, that his wife found out about it from her therapist, who found out about it from his therapist. In his next session he is pissed at his therapist, who reminded him that he agreed to this type of disclosure by signing on the dotted line when he entered the program. The clinic makes the argument that the team approach provides accountability. The spouse feels secure about the approach because she doesn't have to live in fear questioning whether he is cheating on her. She believes that her spouse is being "monitored" and that any slips of sexual sobriety will be reported to her.

> Learning how the system works, the sex addict may conclude that he is better off gaming the system than being honest with his individual therapist. He talks a good game to his therapist, having learned how to lie to his partner. His spouse then lives with a false sense of belief in his fidelity. If she discovers his continuing infidelity, she will have another entity to be angry with: the treatment

clinic or therapist. She chose this treatment option for her partner because of her belief that its "team approach" would keep her safe, and likes the idea that if he cheats again she will know about it.

The important caveat here is that the partner will only learn about the slip if he is open with his therapist, and he may be open only until he learns the consequences of disclosure. One way to get around this problem is to refer the sex addict to an individual therapist outside the clinic who has a very specific confidentiality agreement with the patient. In essence, it says, "I will report back to your wife's therapist and group therapist only that you are attending sessions with me and whether or not I think you are making progress in treatment. I will not discuss with anyone if you have a slip and act out sexually."

Of course, an outside referral may not be necessary if the clinic therapist decides to utilize a similar approach. Alternatively, the clinic may recommend a structured "full disclosure" exercise, as outlined by Corley and Schneider (2002). "Practice guidelines outlined for clinicians include obtaining and gathering history, the importance of establishing goals with clients, timing of disclosure, how much to disclose, and how to disclose. Other ethical situations and steps to rebuild relationships are discussed. Consent for release of information form dictates specifically what type of information will be shared."

Full disclosure may initially seem preferred to the betrayed partner. She may even search for a program that has disclosure of slips in sexual sobriety built in the program. These programs may in fact market themselves in this way to appeal to betrayed partners. Upon further reflection, it may be in her best interest if her partner can freely disclose slips to his therapist without negative repercussions. He may continue to act out, but at least he is discussing it with someone who is there to help him accomplish the goal of sexual sobriety and recovery. Failure to make progress in treatment *can* be disclosed to the partner, who may or may not be surprised. If she is surprised, it can provide the therapeutic leverage needed to make the individual therapy more effective. For example, ITC, an outpatient treatment program in northern California, suspends group therapy if a member does not appear to be motivated to make progress. Then there is open discussion about it. If the member continues to fail to make progress, he may be asked to leave the group, then faced with the prospect of answering his partner's question: "Why are you home? Don't you have your group on Tuesday night?"

Splitting Within the Treatment Team

The ideal treatment team consists of skilled clinicians who generally trust the integrity of their fellow team members and are familiar with how they work. For example, it's possible for a psychodynamic individual therapist to respect the cognitive behavioral approach used by the group therapist because they have worked together successfully in the past. They appreciate each other's strengths and weaknesses and, if a problem arises, they are not afraid to have a frank discussion about a mistake that has been made. They also recognize how the work of one supports the work of the other. If a patient tells his individual therapist he wants to quit group, the next question the therapist generally asks is whether he has discussed it with his group. The same happens if a patient tells his group he wants to quit individual therapy. The two therapists are aligned in supporting the goals of intimacy, which require honesty and openness.

In less-than-ideal circumstances, treatment team members may be suspicious or even contemptuous of one another. This leaks out from the therapist to the patient and reinforces the splitting of the patient, who may want to see his individual therapist as favored over the couples therapist or his spouse's therapist. Briefly, splitting is a psychological defense that serves to simplify the world. Person A is good, and Person B is bad. It's fairly simple. In popular language, such "black and white thinking" involves saying things like, "This person doesn't seem to be able to see things in shades of gray." The person who sees himself as "hero or zero" has difficulty seeing himself as someone who is just OK. He is unable to find the middle ground. He can't seem to see himself—or those around him—as "having good traits and bad traits." They are either "all good" or "all bad."

Most experienced therapists are aware of the possibility that they may be split by the patient into two groups: the good therapists and the bad therapists. When a patient praises us but criticizes the therapist who works with her acting out partner, we need to take note. Does the discordance make sense? Does she have legitimate grievances? If the answer to either of these questions is "yes," the concerns need to be explored and brought to the attention of the other therapist if confidentiality allows. If instead her concerns are vague and seem unsubstantiated, some splitting may be happening. "My husband's therapist has been working with him for six months and he is still hung up on his girlfriend" sounds like splitting; it also sounds like she doesn't understand the therapeutic process.

Splitting in Everyday Life

Practitioners who embrace OR theory or have a psychodynamic orientation generally understand splitting to be a primitive defense. Only the more primitive (disturbed) patients are believed to utilize it as a defense. We have a slightly different notion about splitting. Though we think of ourselves as relatively healthy emotionally, under the right circumstances we use a splitting defense on a fairly regular basis. In fact, many people do it almost every night when watching the news. Our cable news networks encourage us to split, gathering data that support our worldview. If we switch channels to a network on the opposite end of the political spectrum, the broadcasters may present "evidence" supporting a completely different worldview. (Notice the quotation marks? The author's splitting is showing!) One channel says that the president is all good and the other says he is all bad. That's the bottom line.

When emotions run high, it's only human to see no good in the person who has pissed us off. When an idiot on the freeway is texting on his phone and drifts across the lane line, dangerously close to scraping the side of our car, he becomes a self-centered narcissistic asshole. We can make no allowance for the fact that his friends and family know him as a genuinely kind, compassionate, and thoughtful person. He is demon spawn and deserves to die in the slowest and most intensely painful way imaginable. It brings us great relief to speculate on what methods might be chosen by a creative sadist (who we would like to enlist in this cause). In an alternate fantasy, the front of our car might be mounted with a rocket-propelled grenade launcher that could take him out at a moment's notice. We have come to the conclusion that even the healthiest individual is capable of splitting under conditions of extreme stress. Knowing this about ourselves allows self-reflection when we find ourselves feeling angry with the other members of the treatment team.

Clinicians should be concerned about splitting defenses utilized by their patients. When multiple therapists are involved in a case, a patient may pick their favorite. One becomes good and the rest become bad. What concerns us more is that clinicians, like politicians, are also capable of splitting, and might not even try to see the other side of a problem.

> I remember working with a man who was concurrently in group therapy with a therapist unfamiliar to me. I was attempting to help him identify his unmet needs that were leading him to act out sexually (generally one of my primary goals in my work with sex addicts). The group therapist had a very different clinical orientation. He used a traditional addiction model that focused on recovery behaviors, and he assigned workbooks to participants. You could identify his approach as "manualized." During a group session, when my patient reported new insights he had gained from individual therapy, the therapist responded in a dismissive tone, "your individual therapist must be a navel gazer." For this therapist, looking inward in the way valued by a psychodynamic therapist appeared to be a waste of time. It delayed the "real" work of changing behaviors. I guess he was right. I am a navel gazer and I tend to want another navel gazer when I choose a therapist for myself. I want them to be doing everything they can to understand their vulnerabilities and strengths. I want them to know themselves and understand their own motivations. To achieve this, they need to be willing to gaze at their navel. Navel-gazing (introspection) provides a person with something that will outlast the episode of treatment.

Competition Among Therapists

In the San Francisco Bay Area, there are more therapists per square mile than probably just about anywhere in the worlds, it seems, other than perhaps New York City and Los Angeles, so it is not uncommon for therapists to see one another as competitors. Animosity can arise when a patient decides to terminate therapy with one clinician to begin therapy with another. Strong feelings are stirred up in the therapists who fall out of favor and hear their clients describing the brilliance of the new favorite.

For example, a couple I recently treated was recovering from an affair. In this case, I became the "good" therapist. The husband would tell me at least one time during each session how much better I was than their last three couples' therapists. I found myself wondering how much longer my favored status would last. When would the couple terminate therapy with me to take up with another "better" therapist?

In a 1994 article for the *American Journal of Psychotherapy*, Arthur Lazarus (1994) described the development of competition and contempt:

> Tension among the psychiatrist, therapist, and primary-care physician may breed competition and contempt unless working alliances are developed. Alliances may be established in many ways, for example, through meetings, telephone calls, and letters. Personal familiarity is often a critical factor in establishing professional alliances, important dimensions may include knowledge of a colleague's competence, respect for his or her integrity, and personality style. . . . Personal relationships form the foundation for referrals and exchange of clinical information. In this context, however, competition between disciplines concerning issues related to turf and self-esteem often arise. (p. 605)

CASE ILLUSTRATION: KEVORK AND SHANNON

Kevork and Shannon called me to arrange for couples therapy after being referred by an outpatient sex addiction clinic. They are a young professional couple in their early 30s with two toddlers at home, a boy and a girl. Her family lives locally and provides daycare for the children. She is a pediatrician and he is a physicist at a national laboratory that does work for the defense department. His family is Armenian and he is the third generation in the United States. She is a first-generation immigrant from Ireland who came to the United States with her parents and younger brother when she was 10 years old. They come to therapy with the complaint from Shannon that Kevork compulsively masturbates to pornography. Discovery occurred six months earlier. Shannon was disturbed at her husband's lack of interest in sex with her, and during a heated conflict, he revealed that he frequently masturbated with pornography online, daily and sometimes multiple times per day. She eventually gave him an ultimatum: He needed to seek help or she would leave him. He was invested in saving his marriage, so they both went to an intake appointment. He agreed to participate in individual and group therapy with two different therapists. She chose individual and group therapy for partners of sex addicts with two different therapists (no overlap between his and her therapists).

Having the same individual and group therapist is not necessarily contraindicated in this type of work, but there may be drawbacks. If material is shared in individual therapy and then intentionally not discussed in group therapy because, in the patient's words, "I already spoke about it and didn't need to talk about it again," it can lead to deadness in the group process. In addition, it may be easier to share something in individual therapy than in group therapy. Exposure to the therapist may be easier than exposure to a therapist plus, say, seven group members. In this situation, the therapist ideally would talk with the patient about how it might be beneficial to overcome reticence to speak about the issue in group.

On the flip side, the patient might speak about feelings toward other group members in individual therapy. Again, the therapist should explore barriers to discussing the feelings in the group. In a facilitated group process cross-talk (speaking directly to another member of the group) is generally encouraged because it enlivens and deepens the sharing and makes possible a degree of intimacy that promotes growth. In contrast, 12-step programs discourage cross-talk. However, even though it is discouraged in 12-step group meetings, cross-talk often takes place following group sessions during periods of conversation and fellowship.

One practical concern when a group therapist is also the individual therapist involves confidentiality. In the most beneficial arrangement, the therapist agrees not to share information from the individual session in the group session. For the patient this provides a sense of safety and a feeling of individual initiative and control of treatment. However, it may be difficult for the therapist to recall what is shared in individual versus group contexts and there may be slipups or mistakes. This can be an especially big headache if the therapist sees multiple members of the group individually. Another option is to consider disclosures in individual or group therapy fair game for discussions in the other format. Of course, this may cause the patient to be extra cautious about what is shared, because they may not be ready for full disclosure.

Another difficulty may arise when there is one therapist for both therapeutic modalities. What if Patient A is having real difficulty with Patient B in group? Suppose you, the reader, see both Patient A and B in individual and group therapy. Patient A really dislikes Patient B and Patient B wants to be friends with Patient A. (This scenario assumes that outside contact between group members is encouraged. It is discouraged in some group processes, but is generally supported in a recovery program.) Patient B discloses her interest in friendship to you, but you know from her sessions that Patient A really dislikes and perhaps has contempt for Patient B. How do you support Patient B in navigating the issue? What if Patient B reaches out to Patient A in a gesture of friendship and is flatly rejected and wounded? Say that discussion in group therapy reveals that Patient A has discussed her dislike of Patient B extensively in her individual therapy. Patient B may be angry at you for not protecting her from potential rejection. Patient A may also be upset at you if she feels that you encouraged Patient B to reach out to her. In your defense, you had good boundaries and acted with professional integrity in safeguarding the content of each patient's disclosures. An appropriate way to deal with this might be to help Patient B explore how she would know if her desire for friendship with Patient A were mutual, but such arrangements will have complications and may be as varied as the individuals involved. It could also be argued that this situation can arise in any individual therapy.

> I recently became aware that two of my patients are good friends. I didn't know this at the outset of treatment, but when one person was discussing the other it became apparent. I couldn't disclose this to either patient without violating confidentiality. Eventually, they discovered it on their own as they discussed their therapy with each other. They were shocked and bewildered to discover that they shared the same therapist, and each of them brought it up during a session. I couldn't confirm or deny the truth of their discovery, of course. I merely commented that "This kind of situation does happen from time to time and I realize it can be uncomfortable when it does." I added that the important thing is that they feel free

to discuss their feelings about this discovery and explore how it affects their psychotherapeutic process. Going forward, each patient tended to speak less about the other one than they did prior to this discovery. They each wondered what the other may have said about them in treatment. This kind of situation, if navigated well, may not necessarily interfere with either treatment. If, however, the primary goal of either patient is to be able to process their friendship with the other patient, it could present a problem. They may find themselves constricted emotionally about this exploration. If that is the case, it might make sense to encourage a referral to another therapist. Fortunately, this was not the case with these two patients; in fact, each seems to be doing very well in their work with me.

Kevork had three therapists involved in his case. I was his couples therapist and he had a group therapist and an individual therapist. I chose to have fairly limited contact with his individual therapist, even though he provided a full consent for release of information between us. I made a judgment that protecting his confidentiality in individual treatment was paramount for him. If he had a slip, I felt that it would be best if it arose in the context of his couples therapy with me, not as a disclosure from his individual therapist. I shared with both Kevork and Shannon my ideas about the consent and my decision to primarily have contact with his group therapist. However, even if disclosure of a slip was made in group I would not bring it into couples therapy. In fact, I let the group therapist know that I didn't want to know about slips. This put me in a situation similar to Shannon. If I suspected by any other means (such as Kevork's behavior, including interest in sexual relations with his wife) that a slip happened, I would explore the issue in front of Shannon. I asked questions such as "How do each of you feel about the decreased frequency of sex?" and "What does it bring up for you?"

This approach seemed to work well for this couple, but there was one disclosure from the group therapist, a friend of mine who disclosed the information to me during a walk one day, that I did bring into the couple's treatment. In addition to being a physicist, Kevork is an accomplished guitarist. During his years in high school and college, he played in bands at small venues. As often happens in life, he got busy with work

> and family and rarely played anymore. During an especially difficult time in his relationship with his wife, he wrote a song about his love for her. One day he brought his guitar to group and sang the song for the members. The group therapist told me that there was not a dry eye in the room. The group was very moved by the melody and the lyrics. Group members asked if he had shared the song with his wife, and he apparently replied that he had not. I considered whether or not to bring this into the couples therapy and decided that it would be useful to do so. In the next session, I "outed" Kevork in front of his wife. She seemed acutely interested, and we discussed why he hadn't shared the song with her. I took a risk. If I had asked him if it was OK to discuss something he shared with his group that week, that might have put him on the spot. I could have called him, but I prefer not to communicate with individuals separately during couples therapy. Here's another option. I could have mentioned that his group therapist shared something he did which moved the other members, and suggest that it could be helpful to share it with his wife. There are numerous ways I could have dealt with this situation, so perhaps the proof is in the pudding. It actually went well, so in hindsight my intuition proved useful.

He said he didn't feel safe sharing it because she had been angry at him at the time. We explored the sense of emotional danger (i.e., fear of rejection of his softer, loving feelings toward her) and I wondered what might make it feel safer. Because Shannon seemed quite curious about the song and expressed interest in hearing it, Kevork felt more comfortable and agreed to share it with her. In the following session he reported that he had played the song for her at home and brought the lyrics to share with me. It was quite beautiful and heartfelt and served as a wonderful illustration of how, at times, it was easier for Kevork to love Shannon at a distance, to discuss things in his group but not with her. The risks of intimacy scared him. Pornography felt quite safe to him because he could feel and fantasize about love at a distance without exposure to rejection. This helped shift the emotional tone of their relationship. Shannon was able to say that her anger was due to her loneliness. She wanted to connect with him, but he stayed safe and kept his distance from her. She did the same because she also feared rejection. She was able to ask that he make more spontaneous connections with her, be courageous at those moments when he wanted to connect, and take the initiative in reaching out to her emotionally and sexually. As I looked back at the disclosure from the couples therapist, I realized that the disclosure of the song to me by his group therapist only took place because of the friendship between Kevork's group therapist and me. Picking up the phone to call another therapist may sound easy. However, collaboration is often difficult and time-consuming.

> I work primarily during the day, and it's not unusual for me to have eight back-to-back patient sessions. Five or six is a more manageable number, but it doesn't always work that way. It is very difficult for another therapist to reach me during the day unless we prearrange a consultation a week or so in advance. On the flip side, many of my colleagues work in the evenings to accommodate their patients' work schedules, and most group work takes place evenings or Saturdays. As mentioned, I happened to be friends with Kevork's group therapist. One of the things we do together is go for a walk and have coffee on Sunday mornings. We both need the exercise and appreciate the fellowship.

Having a friend who is a colleague has other benefits that are more personal in nature.

> Openly expressing feelings about their job and obtaining a social support network may lead to a reduction in or prevention of therapists' feelings of burnout. Further suggestions include engaging in physical exercise. (Rosenberg, 2006, p. 89)

Colleagues who share several patients in common benefit from the opportunity to collaborate.

> Even though it's not the stated purpose of our morning coffee, we do occasionally discuss patients we have in common if we have their consent, which we had from Kevork and Shannon. In this case, something happened during an informal consultation that amplified the power and meaning of the work. What happened in Kevork's group impacted his group therapist, and in sharing it with me it also impacted me. I brought it into the couples work so it could have an impact on the relationship between Kevork and Shannon.

The Blind Men and the Elephant

We all know the story of the blind men and the elephant. Each of them touches a different part of the elephant, so they come up with very different descriptions of the same animal. The leg feels like a tree trunk, the trunk feels like a large rubber hose, and the tail feels like a snake. In the same way, discussions with different therapists about a patient can be an illuminating experience. We each attend to different parts of the patient. There are questions that we typically ask, and things we remember from interviews. The things we attend to probably have a lot to do with our own values and formative life experiences. There are pieces we relate to and pieces we tend to forget. It's like going to a memorial service where the guests speak about their memories of the deceased. It usually reveals different perspectives on the loved one.

CASE ILLUSTRATION: STEVEN

At my father's memorial I got to hear who he was to his lifelong friends. I didn't have this particular perspective because I was his son and knew him only as my father. At that time I was collaborating with a colleague about a man named Steven who I was seeing in couples therapy. I gained a very interesting perspective from his individual therapist that was very different from the one I had in the couples work. In couples therapy Steven would often raise his voice when he and his wife had arguments. At times he seemed overly aggressive verbally toward his wife, and a bit of a bully. When I mentioned this to his individual therapist, he shared that Steven was terrified of his wife. Steven felt that she often shredded him with her words and viewed himself as vulnerable and defenseless to her attacks. This was extremely helpful information. I didn't need to reference the consultation with the individual therapist during a couples session, but it shifted something in me. I created space within my representation for Steven's vulnerability and could eventually speak to it. He wasn't one to easily show vulnerability but the insight I got from his other therapist allowed me to explore it in couples therapy. I said, "I notice that your voice becomes louder in a way that could be perceived as aggressive, but I wondered if you might in fact feel quite vulnerable when you speak of important things to your wife. Maybe you get loud to protect yourself from that vulnerability much like one might do when making a preemptive strike, fearing that she is about to strike you." When Steven confirmed his fears, his wife softened, and the dynamic shifted completely. She had not been aware of the fear beneath the surface. As a child he had been severely beaten by his mother. Exploring his fear of his wife led him to remember these events, so he was able to share the memories with her and she approached him with more compassion.

Physician, Heal Thyself

When we collaborate with other clinicians, we become aware of our own biases. If we are to be effective in our work, such knowledge is essential. These collaborations force us to grow and self-reflect. It's also one of the implicit rewards in our work with patients. Working with different clients who have unique personalities forces us to stretch and learn something new about ourselves. In exploring the subjective experience of the healing professional, Santorelli (1999) candidly revealed that he often received as much from his patients as they received from him. In the summary of his book he states,

> Perhaps our real work, whether offering or seeking care, is to recognize that the healing relationship—the field upon which patient and practitioner meet—is, to use the words of the mythologist Joseph Campbell, a "self-mirroring mystery"—the embodiment of a singular human activity that raises essential questions about self, other, and what it means to heal thy self.

In the context of the healing relationship, the injunction "heal thyself" applies not just to physicians but to patients as well.

> Personally, to stay balanced in this profession, I (Joe Farley) am involved in a weekly leaderless men's group composed of seven psychotherapists in the San Francisco Bay Area. I have been a member of the group for over 25 years. This group of therapists began in the 1980s at the time of the men's movement in the Bay Area. Leaders in the movement, like Bly (1990), were encouraging men to gather regularly with other men. I have found it one of the

most enriching growth experiences I've had, on par with—but different from—individual therapy. I highly recommend that all therapists find a safe peer support group.

Professional Burnout

Collaboration with other professionals is not just useful for the patient. It is also helpful for the therapist as a protection against burnout. Nayoung (2010) conducted a meta-analysis of studies on burnout among mental health professionals, and found the following:

> Age was the most significant indicator regarding all three dimensions of burnout: emotional exhaustion, depersonalization, and level of personal accomplishment . . . as mental health professionals get older, they are less likely to experience emotional exhaustion . . . mental health professionals are likely to accumulate life experience with emotional maturity that serves as a coping strategy as they get older. . . . We could conclude that younger mental health professionals are more vulnerable to burnout, possibly because of lack of experience that only comes with age. Therefore, it may be more important for younger mental health professionals to secure support and mentoring from their colleagues. This is also important for those with fewer years of work experience, especially if they are to avoid depersonalizing their clients. (p. 90)

Some of the most satisfying experiences we've had in our work have been collaborations with other professionals. Seeing these as a means of marketing and self-promotion sucks the joy out of the experience. If instead these are viewed as opportunities for personal and professional growth, they become connections to look forward to.

12-Step Programs and a Higher Power

Exploring the idea of a higher power in addiction recovery may seem out of place in a book on psychodynamic and psychoanalytic psychotherapy like this one. However, the notion of a higher power is essential to 12-step programs for addiction recovery.

AA, the original 12-step program that led the way, has branched out into programs that address multiple types of addictions, including narcotics, marijuana, sex, gambling, food, work, shopping, hoarding, codependency, and many more. Over 30 different 12-step programs exist today. Any discussion of coordinated treatment modalities for sex addiction must certainly include 12-step programs, most of which utilize the 12 steps and 12 traditions of AA. At AA's request, portions of their literature are read at the meetings of several different 12-step programs. AA literature has become, if you will, part of the official canon.

The 12 steps of AA are described in "the big book," as it is commonly referred to by people in the programs. The first three steps are as follows:

> Here are the steps we took, which are suggested as a program of recovery:
>
> 1. We admitted we were powerless over alcohol—that our lives had become unmanageable.
> 2. Came to believe that a Power greater than ourselves could restore us to sanity.
> 3. Made a decision to turn our will and our lives over to the care of God as we understood Him. (Alcoholics Anonymous, 1939, pp. 59–60)

The big book was authored by AA founder Bill W. He was an end-stage alcoholic close to death when he ended up at the Charles B. Towns Hospital for Drug and Alcohol Addictions in New York City. This was where the wealthy came to dry out, including American millionaires, European royalty, and oil sheiks from the Middle East. Bill's wife was told to prepare for his death, and that his case was hopeless, by William Duncan Silkworth, MD, a preeminent addiction specialist of his time.

After he was discharged from the hospital, Bill W. had a spiritual awakening when an old drinking buddy, "Ebby" Thacher, dropped by his house and shared how he himself had managed to get and stay sober with the help of God. Bill W. was surprised to see Ebby doing so well, but he was an atheist and was uneasy about any talk of God. His friend insisted that he could use the concept of a higher power of his own creation to the same effect, an approach more palatable to him. Bill W. got sober and helped others do the same just as his friend had done for him. He shared with them a message of hope about how a power greater than himself had saved him from alcoholism and certain death and told them that a higher power based on their own beliefs could save them from their alcoholism in the very same way. He realized that his own recovery depended entirely on helping others get sober. When he started to have cravings, he would go to bars and find alcoholics to talk to and help assist him in maintaining his sobriety. After a movement sprang up around his efforts, which he called Alcoholics Anonymous,[1] he demonstrated considerable success in treating "hopeless" alcoholics.

Bill returned to Dr. Silkworth, who was surprised and amazed to see him alive and doing well, and Bill requested the opportunity to work with some of the doctor's alcoholic patients. Dr. Silkworth had firmly believed that Bill would die soon after discharge from the hospital. What surprised Silkworth even more was his patients' favorable responses to Bill's message. Bill shared the story of his spiritual awakening and how belief in a higher power was essential for alcoholics, who had demonstrated that they did not have the power to heal themselves. Bill asked Dr. Silkworth to write a letter to be included in the foreword of "the big book." The doctor did write a letter but did so anonymously; he would have lost considerable status as a leader in the field of addiction if he advocated treatment that relied on belief in a higher power. In later editions, after AA had become widely established and had demonstrated success, Dr. Silkworth modified the letter and allowed his name to be revealed. Here's what he included in the latest edition:

> The subject presented in this book seems to me to be of paramount importance to those afflicted with alcoholic addiction. . . . I say this after many years' experience as Medical Director of one of the oldest hospitals in the country treating alcoholic and drug addiction. (Alcoholics Anonymous, 2001, p. xxvii)

In this later edition, Dr. Silkworth described the difficulty of treating alcoholics. For clinicians then and today, it can be a

---

1. Bill W.'s AA was based loosely on a fellowship of his time known as the Oxford Group.

soul-crushing experience. Many therapists have been humbled by the powerful grip of addiction on their patients.

> Men have cried out to me in sincere and despairing appeal: "Doctor, I cannot go on like this! I have everything to live for! I must stop, but I cannot! You must help me!" Faced with this problem, if a doctor is honest with himself, he must sometimes feel his own inadequacy. Although he gives all that is in him, it often is not enough. One feels that something more than human power is needed to produce the essential psychic change. Though the aggregate of recoveries resulting from psychiatric effort is considerable, we physicians must admit we have made little impression upon the problem as a whole. Many types do not respond to the ordinary psychological approach. (Alcoholics Anonymous, 2001, p. xxix)

Dr. Silkworth went on to describe what seemed to him to be an essential element of successful treatment:

> Frothy emotional appeal seldom suffices. The message which can interest and hold these alcoholic people must have depth and weight. **In nearly all cases, their ideals must be grounded in a power greater than themselves**, if they are to re-create their lives. (Alcoholics Anonymous, 2001, p. xxviii, bold added)

Bill W. began the first draft of the big book in 1938, the same year that Sigmund Freud, a Jew, left Austria for the United Kingdom to avoid persecution by the Nazis. Freud died in the United Kingdom the very next year in 1939, the same year that the big book was published. Sigmund Freud, recognized as the father of psychoanalysis, held views on religion and God that were very different from those of Bill W.

Freud's Views of God and Religion

While Freud seemed fascinated with the notions of God and religion, he believed man's interest in them to be primarily defensive. When he identified himself more as a Jew than a German, he was valuing culture over religion.

> Freud maintained his stance as an uncompromising atheist, the stance he is best known for down to the present. In "The Future of an Illusion," he described belief in God as a collective neurosis: he called it "longing for a father." (Edmundson, 2007, p. 1)

In his *New Introductory Lectures on Psychoanalysis*, Freud (1933) wrote, "religion is an illusion and it derives its strength from its readiness to fit in with our instinctual wishful impulses." In his view, God was entirely a figment of man's imagination, and when man looked to the heavens for answers, he was creating God in his own image to address unacknowledged wishes and desires. "I believe that a large portion of the mythological conception of the world which reaches far into the most modern religions is nothing but psychology projected into the outer world" (Freud, 2017, p. 1125).

Toward the end of his life, Freud's views on God and religion shifted slightly. He began to see a useful purpose in man's musings about God. Rather than thinking of God as a crutch that man created, he began to consider value in man's quest for the mysterious God.

> In his last completed book, "Moses and Monotheism," something new emerges. There Freud, without abandoning his atheism, begins to see the Jewish faith that he was born into as a source of cultural progress in the past and of personal inspiration in the present. Close to his own death, Freud starts to recognize the poetry and promise in religion. (Edmundson, 2007, p. 1)

Perhaps in part due to his fast-approaching death, Freud began to consider that a belief in an unseen God somehow added depth to an individual's life. It freed a person from the tangible and concrete to ponder the mystery of life. It allowed a person to think symbolically and to search the depth of their own soul in a new way, privileging the man who had faith over the one who didn't.

> Suffering badly from cancer of the jaw, Freud offers another perspective on faith. He argues that Judaism helped free humanity from bondage to the immediate empirical world, opening up fresh possibilities for human thought and action. He also suggests that faith in God facilitated a turn toward

> the life within, helping to make a rich life of introspection possible. (Edmundson, 2007, p. 1)

This later view of Freud approaches Masterson's concept of the real self. Masterson believed that the real self was the sum total of the intrapsychic self plus object representations. These representations are revealed only in the course of deep introspection, a path that was, for many, the road not taken. Deep introspection can happen in psychotherapy and psychoanalysis. But these aren't the only ways that someone can realize the potential of the real self. Creative pursuits require intense discipline and fortitude and can help a person discover what is in the depths of their own mind and soul. Masterson uses the example of author Thomas Wolfe as an individual who had the courage to address his demons. Wolfe, like many of the patients Masterson wrote about, utilized the acting-out defenses of drinking and womanizing,

> showing poor reality perception, weak impulse control, little frustration tolerance, and vague ego boundaries. . . . He was having enormous difficulty activating his talent and creativity on his own because of his abandonment depression. (Masterson, 1985, p. 152)

He suffered severe abandonment depression when he traveled abroad and was quite desperate. He met a woman who helped soothe some of his suffering. Perhaps the relationship with her helped him heal some of his developmental trauma. Perhaps she helped him achieve what we might refer to today as an earned secure state of mind concerning attachment (Main, 2000).

> But he did not give up, he kept at it, and suddenly he began to write like a madman, tranced in a hypnosis by whose fatal and unsatiated compulsions he was forced without will to act. The words were wrung out of him in a kind of bloody sweat. He wrote them with his heart, his brain, his sweat, his guts, his blood, his spirit. They were wrenched out of the last secret source and substance of his life and in them was packed the whole image of his bitter homelessness, his intolerable desire, his mad longing for return. They were all there without coherence, scheme or reason. (Nowell, 1960, pp. 94–95, as cited in Masterson, 1985)

This type of transformation is not uncommon among sex addicts. The following case illustrates this principle of transformation.

CASE ILLUSTRATION: JEREMY

Jeremy was a 47-year-old psychologist in treatment for sex addiction. Although happily married, he was in the habit of acting out with sex workers. He had started attending SAA meetings about four months prior and had been in sobriety for just as long. He worked with a sponsor who he spoke to for 15 minutes once or twice a week.

Jeremy: There was this guy, at the last meeting I went to. He had a physically abusive father and his mother was an alcoholic. In fact, his father beat his older brother to death in front of his eyes when he was only five years old. They never talked about it. They said he got sick. His dad used to bring home prostitutes and this guy remembers being confused but intrigued by these women. So of course, this guy was acting out with prostitutes just like I did.

Therapist: That's a pretty incredible story. How did it impact you?

Jeremy: So . . . I started bawling. Tears are running down my face and I'm looking down at my hands folded in my lap for the longest time. I'm kind of embarrassed. When he's done sharing I look up and there are several other guys who have been crying. . . . I know this guy. I've made program calls to him. I never knew his story in this much detail. Based upon his early life this guy should be totally fucked up. This guy really should be fucked up. But he's not. I know this guy. He's a great guy. He's kind and considerate. As I'm sitting there in this meeting the thought occurs to me, I've never helped anyone heal in my practice to the degree this guy shows in his life. I start to feel really inadequate, or maybe humbled is a better word.

Therapist: Yes, I think I understand what you are saying.

Jeremy: But then I realize, this is the God part of the program. This is the higher power thing. I don't know how else to account for it.

Therapist: Hmm. Have you seen that before in program?

Jeremy: You're talking about me aren't you? [Smiles wryly]

Therapist: I admit I was thinking of you but I'm wondering if you have seen others heal in ways that seem beyond human power.

Jeremy: I was actually thinking at that meeting that as I looked around at the other guys, there were several people who seem to have had similar miracles. This was the most dramatic, but there is a lot of recovery in that meeting. It's my favorite for that reason. The stories are very inspiring.

Therapist: So how are you feeling about the work that you are doing with people? I think you said you felt humbled?

Jeremy: I know that I have helped people with addiction, but as I look back the ones who do best have been willing to invest themselves in a 12-step program. That's the humility part. Even though I'm a sex addict and alcoholic and I understand addiction I can't give them all they need. And then there is the God part, or the higher power part. You know, I think that's the special sauce . . .

There is about a two-minute pause and he starts to tear up.

Jeremy: What the fuck. I don't believe in God! But I'm having this feeling I used to have as a little boy going to church at special times. It felt like something greater than me was at work here. I even feel embarrassed to talk about it . . . why . . . I don't know. This is what I felt in that meeting . . . I wonder if those times I have made a real connection with my clients . . . I had this thought that maybe it's the higher power in me and the higher power in my client making some kind of connection. It sounds kind of stupid when I say it.

Therapist: It sounds like you are trying to describe a very meaningful . . . let's say . . . spiritual experience. Words don't always suffice but in addition to the difficulty of finding the words to describe it you also feel self-conscious. Maybe I and others will see you as this little child in church having this childlike experience. Then to protect yourself it seems like you grabbed the word stupid to describe it. Maybe this was like a preemptive strike because you imagined I was thinking it was a stupid thing so you beat me to it with that label.

Jeremy: Yeah. It is uncomfortable. It feels simple-minded. I called the guy who was qualifying [the featured speaker] and I told him about my experience. I felt a little vulnerable talking to him about it as well but he really seemed to get it. He's not a therapist but he thought my idea of our higher power being a powerful element not only in program but in therapy as well made a lot of sense. He said he has been in therapy for quite a few years also but that it wasn't therapy alone that got him to the place he is today.

You may read this brief exchange and think that we are laying out a case for God as adjunct therapist in the treatment of addiction. It may also seem like the SAA sponsor, along with God, is part of the treatment team. In a sense, this may be the case. However, most of the time the therapist does not collaborate with the sponsor. This is a private domain. The anonymity of 12-step programs is sacrosanct. From time to time a patient may reveal to us experiences that deal with a sponsor, higher power, or program, but we generally leave these subjects to the initiative of the patient to discuss. We might ask about a patient's general experience in a program, but that's usually as far as we probe.

Perhaps as Freud expressed toward the end of his life, we don't have to reify a person's belief in God. Freud didn't necessarily become a believer in a higher power, but he did seem to become a believer in the clinical benefits of belief in a higher power. Belief in a higher power of their own making (and participation in a recovery fellowship) grants a unique advantage to our patients when it comes to battling sexual addiction. It may only be in their minds. Nonetheless, it seems to give them the extra boost they need to achieve a solid recovery.

CHAPTER 7

Couples Therapy

In William Stafford's (1998) poem, "A Ritual to Read to Each Other," he writes, "If you don't know the kind of person I am / and I don't know the kind of person you are / a pattern that others made may prevail in the world / and following the wrong god home we may miss our star." We could analyze the first piece of Stafford's (1998) poem and draw many conclusions. One that seems apparent is that openness and honesty lead to intimacy and help couples avoid the pitfalls of ambiguity. If we don't speak our truth, someone else's truth will prevail.

He goes on to write, "For there is many a small betrayal in the mind, / a shrug that lets the fragile sequence break / sending with shouts the horrible errors of childhood / storming out to play through the broken dike." If one doesn't know one's own truth, childhood trauma will tell its own truth in a way that may not be to our liking. We might get lazy and, not knowing our own truth, let things around us fall where they may.

Stafford finishes the poem with a sad but true statement about how we may really want to arrive at a certain destination in our life but not recognize how far off course we actually are. "And as elephants parade holding each elephant's tail, / but if one wanders the circus won't find the park, / I call it cruel and maybe the root of all cruelty / to know what occurs but not recognize the fact."

We may know this, but may be entirely incapable of acting differently because of the power of the unconscious and our personal history. In extramarital affairs, a person acts out old unconscious relational needs and desires. Then they find themselves lying to their partners, and they may feel they have gotten away with it. When they wake up they find they have fallen into a very deep dark hole.

"And so I appeal to a voice, / to something shadowy, / a remote important region in all who talk: / though we could fool each other, we should consider— / lest the parade of our mutual life get lost in the dark. / For it is important that awake people be awake, / or a breaking line may discourage them back to sleep; / the signals we give—yes or no, or maybe— / *should be clear: the darkness around us is deep.*"

In this chapter we look at some of the many things that can go astray throughout a couple's life. An obvious one for us to explore in a book about sexual addiction and other problems is infidelity.

What do the macaroni penguin, sandhill crane, seahorse, gray wolf, barn owl, shingleback skink, bald eagle, gibbon ape, black vulture, beaver, and swan have in common? Research indicates that all of these mate for life (Nowak, 2019). Should human beings also be included in that list? Ryan and Jetha (2010) argue that this isn't really natural for humans. They think we hold an almost unattainable standard when we expect our spouse to remain faithful throughout our life. Fincham reports that 45–50% of married women and 50–60% of married men cheat on their spouses (Fincham, 2017). Does it make sense to refer to extramarital affairs as pathological, or should we view it, in light of statistics on cheating, as normative? We don't necessarily answer this question for the reader. When a couple comes to us they get to define the problem.

It does seem more difficult for couples to sustain their relationship over the long term these days. During the COVID-19 pandemic, couples initially became closer. For the first time they had an abundance of time together with many working from home. As the pandemic wore on, couples became more and more isolated from their extended families. But such isolation has been going on for a long time. By the time they come to therapy, many couples may have moved three or four times across the country for work or other reasons, and parents and siblings are often scattered across the globe. During the pandemic, couples seemed more isolated than at any other time in recent history. Many people don't have close friends and don't even know their neighbors. As a result, many people have come to expect their partner to be everything for them: best friend, lover, confidant, spiritual adviser, and coparent. Expectations like this of any one person are unreasonable and often lead to disappointment and disillusionment.

Providing a Nonjudgmental Therapeutic Experience for Both Addict and Partner

One of the challenges for a couples therapist is to maintain an objective, neutral perspective. This is nearly impossible. Sometimes the therapist is pulled to identify with the betrayed partner. At other times, they identify with the unfaithful partner. Couples therapy becomes an emotional tug of war in which each partner implicitly tries to curry favor with the therapist. They want to know, at least, that the therapist empathizes with their position. Although an admirable goal, objectivity is rarely attained. It's best to acknowledge this and be aware of when you are being pulled toward one patient or the other. A therapist who is planning to work with couples needs to turn inward and examine their own experiences in romantic relationships and how these experiences may affect their attitudes toward struggling couples (Silverstein, 1998). A therapist needs to ask, "Have I ever had a healthy, satisfying romantic relationship?" If not, they may feel that good relationships are impossible, and that cynicism will eventually and inevitably creep into their work. On the other hand, if they have an overly romanticized notion of what a healthy relationship looks like, they may unconsciously hold up a standard that neither they nor their poor clients can ever achieve.

If the therapist has been in a relationship in which their partner cheated, will feelings of hurt and betrayal cause them to be too harsh and critical of the cheater and to identify too much with the partner? If the therapist was the unfaithful one, will they over-identify with the cheater and implicitly blame the partner for not meeting the needs of the one who strayed?

These questions should be extended to the therapist's family background. If one of the therapist's parents cheated, will they carry a grudge and project their feelings onto the cheating member of the couple? If, as a child, the therapist felt pressured to take over the role of the absent spouse and become overly responsible for emotional support, did they grow to resent the betrayed parent? If the custodial parent was the only one there to absorb the child's anger and resentment, as an adult the therapist might believe that if Mom treated Dad better maybe he wouldn't have cheated, and project blame onto the betrayed partner.

There's a good reason for asking yourself all these questions. Couples therapy is often so emotionally intense—especially where sexual addiction and acting out occurs—that the risk of countertransference acting out (when the therapist acts out intense feelings) is very high. If there was ever a case for a therapist to be fully aware of their countertransference vulnerabilities it is here. Those aspiring to provide couples therapy must be sure that they have thoroughly explored their own family of origin issues as they relate to potential countertransference. Ongoing supervision and collaboration with other clinicians are also highly recommended to help sort out issues as they surface in the work.

CASE ILLUSTRATION: DAN AND VICKIE

Dan and Vickie came to therapy in the aftermath of Vickie's discovery that Dan was having sex with prostitutes, one in particular. These hookups often happened when Dan was out of town visiting his parents and brother. These visits became more and more frequent and lasted longer and longer. He became a regular client of a sex worker who called herself Ginger, and he fell in love with her.

He began to spend full days with her, and they went on some overnight trips together. Vickie noticed the increase in cash withdrawals from the ATM and became suspicious. It all exploded when she found a text message with a heart emoji from Ginger saying that she had really enjoyed their weekend together. When Vickie scrolled down she discovered sexually explicit text messages.

Both Dan and Vickie had been raised in fundamentalist Christian families. She was shocked and disgusted by his behavior, and he was experiencing intense shame at being caught. They had consulted two previous couples therapists without success. Vickie felt that their first therapist—a man—was not sensitive enough to her concerns. Dan believed the same about the second therapist—a woman—and thought she grilled him too much about his affair but was too easy on his wife despite her out-of-control behavior.

Vickie had told their teenage children details about Dan's cheating behavior, and they were hurt and angry at their father. Dan kept trying to get the female therapist to tell Vickie that she was wrong to tell their children about his cheating. She had explained that Vickie needed emotional support and, since he was absent, he left her no option but to turn to other members of her family. Dan was adamant that couple's therapy wouldn't work unless I would side with him on this point, and he blamed Vickie for the deteriorating relationship with his children.

They were embroiled in a nasty fight, and it was clear from the outset of treatment that I was going to have my hands full. Each wanted me to scold the other. Their idea of therapy was for me to be a priest and therapist who would point out the other's sinful wrongdoing and mandate appropriate penance. In their minds, this would involve enumerating sinful deeds, acknowledging debasement, eliciting contrition, and ultimately granting forgiveness. Amazingly, despite the failure of the previous two therapists who followed this strategy, they thought I could be successful doing the same. It's not logical. But couple conflicts rarely are.

Dan proclaimed that Vickie would never forgive him, and Vickie proclaimed that Dan was never contrite in his apologies and requests for forgiveness. Fife (2013) describes the process of forgiveness as including four components: empathy, humility, commitment, and apology. Both Dan and Vickie struggled in all of these domains. Although falling short of a DSM-5 diagnosis, they both have narcissistic tendencies and lived the early decades of their relationship in a kind of fused state with very little differentiation. An assumption of like-mindedness formed the basis of fantasies about their closeness in both family and business matters. They co-owned a successful insurance brokerage business and didn't veer far off the script of their lives as happy couple and business owners. They settled for pseudo-intimacy, as true intimacy would require vulnerability, differentiation, disagreements, and dialogue. Empathy and humility were certainly not either of their strong suits. Vickie's discovery caused an avalanche of feelings: terror, humiliation, disappointment, disillusionment, rage, shame, inadequacy, and despair. Dan felt humiliated, ashamed, guilty, perverse, wretched, angry, sad, inadequate, and panicky. He felt his life, his family, and his business crumbling around him. He felt desperate and powerless to put Humpty Dumpty back together again.

Therapist: [Beginning our first session] Hi, it's nice to meet both of you. I'd like to hear a little bit from each of you about what brings you into couples therapy.

Dan: We've been in therapy twice already. It might speed things up if you could talk to our last therapist and she can fill you in on the details. [He's looking for an easy out here. The last thing he wants to do is have to talk about his affair with a sex worker.]

Therapist: I'm sure it's hard to tell your story all over again, but I'd really like to hear it in your own words if that's OK.

Dan: OK . . . I had an affair but it's over now . . .

Vickie: [Interrupting] Is it really over? [Looking at me] You see, I'm not sure it's over. He's told me it's over at least four or five times now and it always turns out it's not over. And by the way, this affair he refers to, it was with a prostitute! [If it was her intent to shame and humiliate him, she has been entirely successful.] Not only did he cheat on me but he used our money to do it! He bought her jewelry, he wined and dined her. He was the big man.

Dan: [Looking down in shame like a dog that has just been scolded] That's true. But she exaggerates. It hasn't been four or five times.

Vickie: [Loudly] How many times has it been, Dan!? How many times did you swear to me that it was over . . . only for me to find out you were lying again!

Dan: You tell me, you seem to be the one keeping score!

This is not a good start. I can feel myself starting to sweat and my heart is beating a little faster than normal. The tension is so thick in the consulting room that it feels like I need to chew each breath of air before I swallow. I am experiencing a stress response. Under the influence of cortisol and adrenaline, my body is preparing for fight or flight, or maybe freeze.

Some therapists become immobilized in this type of situation. If as children they experienced parents fighting, they may have learned to freeze to avoid detection and stay below the radar. Physiologically this is like pushing the accelerator of a car while standing on the brakes. It's not good for a car, and it's certainly not good for a human being's body, either. Freezing is a parasympathetic brake on the sympathetic fight or flight response (Schore, 2010).

Therapist: [Trying to achieve a neutral tone] I'd really like to be able to help you guys do this differently than you've done it before. My guess is that's why you're here. I know these are very emotional things we are talking about but if you talk over each other, I won't be able to hear you and, more importantly, you won't hear each other. Could we try that again?

Dan: She's right. I told her it was over and it wasn't. More than one time . . . a few times. I just got involved with this person and one thing led to another. It was hard to break it off.

Therapist: Why are you here, Dan?

Dan: I want to see if we can work things out.

Therapist: Work things out?

Dan: I want to see if Vickie can ever forgive me. I don't want a divorce. I wasn't very happy before . . . that's why . . .

Vickie: [Interrupting] He's rewriting history. He certainly seemed happy before. Just ask anyone.

Therapist: [To Dan] Do you know why you weren't happy before?

Dan: We fought all the time. I felt controlled all the time. And Vickie can't stand my family and . . .

Vickie: [Interrupting] Why don't you tell him why, Dan?

Dan: She's never got along with them. My parents feel like she doesn't treat them well and she feels my parents don't treat her well. That's the way it's been for a while now.

Vickie looks like she is about to explode. I realize that I'd better let her speak soon or she won't be able to contain herself and will keep interrupting Dan.

Therapist: Vickie, let's leave this here for now. We can explore it later, but I'd like to hear from you why you are here.

Vickie: [Looking really pissed] Well, Joe, we are here today basically because Dan can't keep his dick in his pants.

Therapist: If that were the only problem, I imagine Dan would be in individual therapy, but you are here with him today. Why's that?

I'm trying to distinguish between individual therapy, where the focus is on one person's problems versus couples therapy, where the couple's relationship is the focus of treatment.

Vickie: He is in individual therapy now! He has been for two years, but it hasn't stopped him from cheating! I don't know what he talks to his therapist about. Obviously, they don't talk about what he should be talking about because he keeps on fucking that bitch. As far as I can tell, therapy hasn't helped him at all. I'm sure he just complains about how horrible I am.

Vickie is really hurt and angry. I'm trying hard to like her, but at the moment I truly don't. If we are to make any progress at all, she will need to be able to go deeper than the anger. Every time she speaks, I see Dan shrinking deeper into his chair. I start to feel protective of him. I decide to go with the anger because I don't see how we can move past it unless we go through it first.

Therapist: Vickie, you sound really angry.

Vickie: You're damn right I'm angry. I'm angry that he lied to me so many times. I'm angry that, when I was desperate to understand what was going on, his family ignored me. They didn't give a damn that I was fighting for my marriage. I'm angry that he broke our marriage vows. He promised me he would never do this. And I'm angry that he seems to blame me for all of it. He never takes any responsibility for himself. I'm the controlling bitch and he's the poor victim.

For the next 10 minutes, she tells me the story of Dan's betrayal. She talks about how his trips to see his parents became longer and longer, and more frequent. She tells me about her serious car accident and the very long recovery. She explains that this was one of the loneliest times of her life. When she needed her husband the most, he disappeared on her. Dan attempts to comfort her by putting his hand on hers, but she pushes it away. Her tone begins with fierce anger and then softens ever so slightly, and I can detect a hint of sadness in her voice.

Vickie: Of all the times I needed him, I needed him then. But he was gone. And then when Jenna [their teenage daughter] heard him talking to his hooker on the phone, my life fell apart. I got his cell phone records and everything became clear. I was a total sucker. I must have been in denial for so long. How could he do that to me? He wouldn't return my calls or pick up when I called, but he was talking to her almost 10 times a day. They would talk for hours.

I mirror her vulnerability as she starts to move from anger to sadness. I can see that Dan is now sitting still in his chair and appears calmer. He still hangs his head, but the nervous foot shaking and looking at the clock have stopped altogether. I ask him how it feels to hear Vickie talk about how it was for her. He seems to struggle with attempts at empathy, but apparently he gives enough that Vickie appears to feel heard by him. I wonder if he has ever heard her tell her story like she did today. Somehow, I can't imagine him sitting still long enough to hear it.

She tells me that, when she tries to initiate a conversation, Dan finds a way to exit. This will become a recurring theme in our sessions. Something interesting happens to me as I listen to Vickie. I start to like her and appreciate what she has been through. The anger had done strange things to her face. As it relaxes, I start to relate to her and identify with her struggles. For the first time, I notice how attractive she is—she's really quite beautiful. It's amazing how a simple change in her state of mind could shift the state of mind of those around her. I imagine that Dan has a similar experience with her. He seems ashamed of himself, but mostly sad for her. He's clearly more open to her now.

Over the next two years, we would explore various themes in therapy. One recurrent theme was trust versus mistrust. When Vickie demonstrated mistrust by commenting that she didn't really know if the affair was over, Dan struggled. This time he really had ended it and expected her to believe him, even though he understood that she would have trouble trusting him. But this awareness of her state of mind was fleeting. When under attack, he would revert to seeing her as withholding, unforgiving, and cruel.

Therapist Neutrality in the Face of Pressure to Take Sides

Both Vickie and Dan desperately wanted the therapist to take their side and felt that empathy toward one was siding against the other. This puts the therapist in an extremely tenuous position. Often it seems like each member of a couple comes intending to obtain a pronouncement from the therapist that they are right and the other partner is wrong. But if they actually got what they wanted, what good would it do? Still, many therapists fall into this trap, and therapy soon ends.

In an attempt to help Dan understand Vickie's attachment insecurity, I would try to get her to explore it in our sessions by describing the pain and despair she felt. She recalled feelings of insanity when she would question him and he gaslit her. Before discovery, she was trying to make sense of the distance in the relationship and his apparent apathy toward her. She had no explanation that made sense, so she questioned herself, fearing that there must be something terribly wrong with her. She thought she was just being paranoid.

She had been in a serious automobile accident a year before Dan's affair and felt entirely alone. She was left with debilitating injuries and was in a full-body cast for months. She had a slow and painful recovery, much of it during the affair. Her teenage children, along with her mother and sister, became her caretakers. This burden affected them deeply and alienated them from Dan. Where was he? Why wasn't he there? They didn't understand why he spent so much time out of town when Vickie needed him most.

She related stories about doctor appointments involving treatment decisions that had to be made and recalled that, even when he was there, he was entirely absent emotionally. This sense of abandonment and betrayal was perhaps more painful than the actual affair. She believed in the oath they made at marriage and that he would be with her in sickness and in health, "til death do you part." The more she relived these experiences and feelings in front of him, the more shame he felt, and the more he distanced himself, both from her and from these painful feelings of having failed his wife in her time of need.

Vickie: It's like you disappear all day and I don't see you or know what you're doing. The few interactions we have are business interactions: "sign this, mail this, make sure you take care of that." You bark orders at me. How am I supposed to feel good about our relationship when this is the only thing you say to me? Then you come home in the evening and you start to feel horny and you want to have sex. You demand it. Then you fuck me and for all I know you are thinking about that woman and just using my body. I start to feel like a whore. You don't make love to me, like I really need now. You just fuck me. But I'm not getting paid. I get nothing. At least she gets money out of the deal. It's like we have no relationship during the day then you fuck me at night like a whore. I can't remember the last time I felt we were making love. All I get is a quick selfish fuck!

Dan: Look, Vickie, I told you I'm sorry. How many times do I have to say it?

Vickie: Then how come I don't feel you are sorry? The words mean nothing if I don't feel you are sincere about it. I don't feel like I have ever had a sincere apology from you. You say sorry to get me off your back . . . it's dismissive. What are you sorry for?

Dan: Don't be ridiculous.

Vickie: I'm serious. What are you sorry for?

Dan: What do you think? For hurting you . . . for the affair. [He seems irritated.]

Vickie: [Looking to me] Do you see what I mean, Joe? Does he seem sorry to you? [She laughs.] It's all bullshit. He's so narcissistic all he thinks of is himself. He just wants the pressure off him. He wants to be relieved of his guilt. I want him to be a man. Step up . . . take responsibility. He just keeps taking the easy way out. I've lost all respect for him. I don't know what happened to the man I married. He's become a wimp.

They are horribly stuck. We've been at this for months, and they don't seem any better. Back before they came to me, they had contacted their health insurance company and were given the names of several local cognitive behavioral therapists. They were told that the efficacy of CBT is supported by empirically based scientific research. Perhaps thinking they should have followed that advice, they start asking me about CBT. What is it? Could it help us? Maybe that will work for them. We are all wondering if I can really help them. She is so angry, and he is so shut down.

Therapist: This is really hard right now. I'm sure you and I would love to think there could be something simple that could really fix this mess that you are in. I'd love that more than anything, but unfortunately, I don't think it exists. At least I'm not aware of it. I think the way to get through it is to stick with it and go right through it. That's how to get beyond it. Unfortunately, there are no short cuts.

What the insurance company had not told them is that insurance companies prefer CBT because it is cheap and quick. The representative had also failed to mention that empirically based research has also demonstrated that people show improvement at the end of CBT but within a short period most of the gains disappear (Shedler, 2010). Psychodynamic approaches have similar success rates, but the gains continue long after treatment ends. There is something lasting that takes place in psychodynamic therapy.

I need to respond to Vickie's question about whether Dan's apology is sincere.

Therapist: I honestly don't know what is in Dan's heart and if his apology is sincere but I'm quite sure that his apology is not helping you feel any better about your relationship. I think he feels your anger and his own shame and guilt and to protect himself from these painful feelings he shuts down and shifts the blame to you. He calls you unforgiving and cold. When he says that it just adds insult to the injury you feel so profoundly. I imagine you might actually feel cold and empty inside and you hope against hope that he can warm you up. You keep hoping he will hear and understand you're hurt. It would be nice to feel in love with him again. When he doesn't see you, your disappointment is so strong that you lash out at him to soothe yourself, but it just makes him close up and you feel more alone.

Vickie [crying]: Being angry is so much easier than being sad. I'd rather fight with him than switch back to feeling pain. I just feel like my heart has been ripped out of my chest. I never imagined this would happen to us. I could never imagine being in this much pain.

I am reminded of the old television ad for Virginia Slims cigarettes. The slogan, repeated by various beautiful women, was, "I'd rather fight than switch." Dan seems to have softened. He reaches over and puts his hand on hers, and she doesn't push him away this time.

Vickie: I really want to get back to where we were before, but I'm losing hope that we can get there.

Dan: I know, me too. I'm so sorry.

This was a good moment. You could feel the ice breaking in the room. Vickie was feeling her pain, and Dan was there with her. When he reached out and grabbed her hand and she didn't pull away, it felt good to both of them to have a moment of real connection. This is how it went for several months. We continued to have breakthroughs in which Vickie would get to her more vulnerable feelings and Dan would open up to her. There began to be softness and kindness between them. As a therapeutic alliance was formed and strengthened over the next several weeks, Dan became more open to my defense interpretations:

> Therapist: I think when Vickie brings up her experience of betrayal and anger it triggers a deep sense of shame within you, and to shield yourself from these feelings you shift the focus onto her shameful behavior. You portray her as a flawed individual without the capacity for forgiveness. This relieves your shame but unfortunately it just inflames her senses of injustice and then she escalates her attempts to demonstrate how uncaring you are. Then you distance to protect yourself and you seem to prove her right in her mind.

Masterson (1976, 1981) referred to this type of intervention as an interpretation of narcissistic vulnerability. The therapist must come from a place of empathic understanding of the patient. He describes how the client focuses on the self and experiences painful affects such as shame or a sense of inadequacy. To protect himself against those feelings he uses one of several types of defenses, such as intellectualization, devaluing, avoidance, or perhaps projecting blame from himself to the other.

Eventually, over time and repeated interpretations of this type, the dynamic shifted slightly. Dan began to allow himself the feelings of guilt as he listened to her recount the history of the affair from her perspective.

> Dan: Every time I hear you talk about this I feel horrible. I feel like the worst person on the planet. And it feels like there is no chance of redemption. I can see I really hurt you and I'm truly sorry about that. I wish I could go back in time and change what I did. I want to take it back. It wasn't worth it. It really wasn't worth it. Let me know how I can help heal this. I want you to feel more secure with me. I wish I could go back to support you with your recovery from your accident when you really needed me. I have made my choice. I want to be with you. You have to believe me.

Countertransference Reactions of the Couples Therapist

It's common for therapists to have negative countertransference to the unfaithful partner and more positive countertransference to the betrayed partner. The therapist's reactions may have a lot to do with prior life experiences from their family or origin or past relationships. The human brain seeks that which is familiar. If a patient has traits that resemble familiar people in the clinician's past it may elicit similar feelings from the past. Our mind attempts to make predictions based upon past experiences and history. Linkages between past and present are constantly being made at an unconscious level. Because this is usually unconscious, the therapist is often surprised when a link between past and present comes into awareness.

In this case my countertransference shifted back and forth. Even though he was quite narcissistic, I initially had more positive countertransference to Dan and negative countertransference to Vickie. Dan didn't interrupt and seemed more self-contained. Vickie was more difficult to manage during our sessions, as she was harsh and her anger was more explosive. Based on the process, this shifted during sessions, but generally this trend continued. I eventually sorted it out. Dan was soft-spoken and deliberate in his words. He also praised me regularly, which usually has a negative effect on me, but because of the contrast with Vickie's harshness and extreme anger, it was easier for me to feel safer with Dan. Because I became aware of this tendency, I deliberately paid attention to my emotional responses in the sessions. When I was able to go beneath the surface with Vickie and hear about her pain, my countertransference shifted. When she was less guarded with anger, I really began to like her.

Intellectually I knew that she was entitled to her anger. In general I don't have trouble with people who are angry unless they start to act it out in a destructive way. Why was I so put off by her anger? Do I get triggered by strong, angry women? So began a period of soul searching. After talking about the issue in my own therapy and discussing it with my colleagues and my wife, I achieved some clarity. I realized that I really do like strong, assertive women. But I don't like it when unleashed anger is directed toward the other in a way that shuts down exploration. I could see that Dan was feeling vulnerable and was not going to expose himself in front of Vickie when she was so angry. If she really wanted to know what led him to seek out prostitutes she would need to contain her anger in a way that would allow him to explore the issue honestly.

CASE ILLUSTRATION: MARY AND STAN, A THERAPEUTIC FAILURE

Vickie and Dan reminded me of another couple I worked with, Mary and Stan. I had a similar discomfort with Mary as I did with Vickie. She was so angry that it was hard to sit with them in the room. Their previous couples therapist had candidly reported disliking her during a brief telephone consultation. The couple had signed a release and asked me to speak with the previous therapist. Stan was passive, and Mary would attack him endlessly. I found myself wanting to protect him. In her rage she would ask him a question and demand an immediate answer. He was obviously scared. How could he answer and be heard? In such cases stepping in and making a process comment would have been the right thing to do, but I didn't. I froze. Stan would tentatively answer her question and she would attack him viciously for his "pathetic" answer. After I finally had enough, I made the following interpretation to Mary.

Therapist: You are so hurt by the affair that you protect yourself with your anger. It's a lot easier to be angry at Stan than to be vulnerable with your sad and hurt feelings. I notice you asked Stan a question and your anger seemed to frighten him. He seemed to feel unsafe with you and dared to give you an answer despite the fear, but you didn't listen to him. You spoke over him when he answered your question. I think he didn't give the answer you wanted so you protected yourself by being angry and attacking him about how he answered you.

This comment could have been helpful, but it wasn't. It was obvious that I was angry with her. I was trying to put her in her place, and she felt it. I was trying to get her to back off, but she was like a dog with a bone. She wouldn't let go.

Mary: Well Stan needs to grow a pair and be able to speak up for himself. He doesn't need you speaking for him.

The angrier she got, the more passive Stan got. She wanted him to be strong, able to handle her anger, and remain in the arena. During the session I got increasingly protective of him. He was passive and I wanted him to speak up.

Eventually Mary angrily stomped out of the session, never to return. This was my fault. I didn't speak from empathy, but from a place of anger deep within myself. I thought she was being abusive toward her husband. It was happening in my office, and I wanted it to stop. Technically, my words were OK. Rather, they were 80% OK. My mistake was reacting too quickly and too emotionally. I'm sure that my own tone was angry and critical, mirroring hers. She saw right through it. I had lost my therapeutic neutrality and was taking sides. I wasn't able to hold onto empathy for Mary and the long period of betrayal she experienced when Stan was having an affair.

Her anger was a reaction to his passivity. Mary wanted to see passion in Stan. They hadn't resumed sexual relations, and she was hungry for it. She was lonely, sexually frustrated, and needed to feel Stan's attraction to her. Granted, she was going about getting it in the wrong way. If she wanted more passion, she needed to approach him in a softer way. All she was doing was scaring him. At times he would get passionate, but it was not exactly what she wanted. She always seemed to need to make him wrong. She would critique his initiative and he would shrink again. He would occasionally fight back like a cornered animal, showing his teeth and claws and escalating his voice to get her to back off, but mostly he was passive and scared.

This raises an interesting question: Is it necessary to like our patients? The answer is complicated. Our colleagues have weighed in on the issue, indicating that they won't treat someone they don't genuinely like. But when you interview a couple or client for the first time, how do you know whether you'll like them? After all, we may like someone in one moment and not in another. To some degree, liking someone is a temporary state of mind. You can like your wife when you're getting along, but not at other moments when you don't appreciate the way she is acting. There are many clients we have liked during the initial interview, but have come to dislike during a particular phase of treatment. Likewise, there are patients who we didn't particularly care for at the outset of treatment, but come to love and admire after their story unfolds.

CASE ILLUSTRATION: THE RETURN OF DAN AND VICKIE

Having learned my lesson with Mary and Stan, I tried to connect with Vickie's vulnerability and encourage her to speak to Dan. As soon as she genuinely trusted that he understood her and was genuinely contrite, she could let up. Eventually she was able to hear from him about the state of mind that led him to go searching elsewhere for connection. Seeking out sex workers felt easy for Dan. He felt he held all the cards. He was paying for a service. He was the customer and the customer is always right. If it didn't go well, there were many other sex workers to choose from. He had met with about five different women until he finally settled on one who could make him feel good about himself. She would tell him what a wonderful man he was, and how unfortunate it was that his wife didn't understand that he was such a great guy, saying, "Something must be wrong with her."

Eventually, Dan and Vickie became able to tolerate each other's feelings, as well as their statements about what they wanted in their relationship. They developed and sustained more empathy toward each other, and increased their tolerance for individuation and differentiation. Eventually, they were able to believe differently about an issue but still respect each other.

Throughout our work, pride decreased and humility increased. They each admitted that they couldn't know the mind of the other unless the other felt safe enough to reveal it. There was more commitment and less withdrawal. Dan answered his phone and let Vickie know his plans for the day. If he caught himself barking orders to her he stopped, but sometimes she still had to remind him. He was eventually able to offer a sincere, heartfelt apology for the affair and his abandonment. Vickie reflected on how she attempted to control situations as a way to contain her anxiety, and became able to stop herself in the process when she noticed it. When she didn't, Dan could let her know he was feeling controlled, and she accepted that feeling. Ultimately, they were able to resume an active sex life. Sometimes it was wild and selfish, and at other times it was more sensitive and fulfilled Vickie's desire to give love and feel loved in return.

Supporting the Emergence of Real Selves in a Relationship

Sometimes an affair is an attempt on the part of the unfaithful partner to repair and heal themselves (Perel, 2017). Or they may feel like something has died inside them and are attempting to bring it back to life. A relationship can become stale and a person can feel unsure about how to reintroduce passion. They may look at their spouse and feel nothing. They may feel passion about a new person that enters their life. They may get excited every time they see or speak with that special coworker or neighbor across the street. They look for more and more opportunities to be in the presence of the other because of how it makes them feel about themself. They feel desirable and attractive. The other seems interested in them and laugh at their humor while their partner is tired of hearing the same old thing. Of course this is appealing. Before long there are lunches scheduled and phone calls or text messages at night when the spouse is asleep. The person feels alive again, rejuvenated and anxiously anticipating the next meeting. This is a far cry from the feeling of boredom the person feels on the drive home from work at the end of the day that was a lot like the day before.

Only toward the end of therapy was Dan able to speak about what was missing for him in his relationship with Vickie. He had several unmet needs he sought to fulfill through the affair. He wanted to feel loved and admired. He wanted a partner who saw the best in him, not the worst. As can often happen in a long-term relationship, he felt taken for granted and was more aware of his wife's irritation with him than her love for him. He found someone else who was interested in him and made him feel valued.

Interestingly, all of what was missing for Dan in their relationship was also what was missing for Vickie. At times it was important for Dan to be explicit with Vickie that, when he discussed his unmet needs, he wasn't blaming Vickie for the affair. He took full responsibility for breaking his wedding vows. This made it easier for Vickie to hear what he needed from the relationship and to want to help fulfill those needs. Through couples therapy, they began to understand each other's needs in a way they hadn't before.

Dan and Vickie had a positive termination. They weren't fixed. All their problems weren't solved. Like all couples, they would continue to bicker at times and feel misunderstood. What they had gained during therapy were the tools to get back in touch. They came to learn that, even though they wanted to protect and defend themselves, they could finally get what they wanted by suspending and containing their emotional responses to listen and hear each other. It was not all of what they wanted, but enough. Our colleague Ken Seider often reminds us of the eternal wisdom of the Rolling Stones (Jagger and Richards, 1969): "You can't always get what you want / But if you try sometimes, well, you might find / You get what you need."

How many times do we hear our patients protest because things are not the way they wish them to be? We are all, no doubt, familiar with the situation in which a patient has a good ending to a course of psychotherapy and says something along the lines of, "You know, I really thought I wanted to this one thing when I started therapy. But over the course of therapy I realized I couldn't have what I wanted. What I got though, was something I needed that was much more meaningful."

References

Ackerman, N. W. (1966). *Treating the troubled family*. Basic Books.

Ainsworth, M., Biehar, M. C., Waters, E., & Wall, S. (1978). *Patterns of attachment: A psychological study of the strange situation*. Erlbaum.

Alcoholics Anonymous. (1939). *Alcoholics Anonymous: The story of how many thousands of men and women have recovered from alcoholism*. Alcoholics Anonymous World Service.

Alcoholics Anonymous. (2001). *Alcoholics Anonymous: The story of how many thousands of men and women have recovered from alcoholism* (4th ed.). Alcoholics Anonymous World Service.

Alexander, R. (1989). Evolution of human intelligence. In R. Alexander (Ed.), *Human social evolution: The foundational works of Richard D. Alexander*. Oxford University Press.

American Psychiatric Association. (2013). *Diagnostic and statistical manual of mental disorders* (5th ed.). American Psychiatric Association.

Arlow, J. (1987). Trauma, play, and perversion. *The Psychoanalytic Study of the Child*, *42*, 3144.

Bader, M. (2009). *Male sexuality: Why women don't understand it—And men don't either*. Rowman & Littlefield.

Bancroft, J., Janssen, E., Strong, D., Carnes, L., Vukadinovic, Z., & Long, J. S. (2003). The relation between mood and sexuality in heterosexual men. *Archives of Sexual Behavior*, *32*(3), 217–230.

Barks, C. (2004). *The essential Rumi*. (New Expanded Ed.). HarperCollins.

Beattie, M. (1978). *Codependent no more*. Hazelden Publishing.

Beebe, B., & Dougherty, K. (2016). *Mother-infant communication: The research of Dr. Beatrice Beebe*. PEP video grants. 1(2), 11. https://pep-web.org/browse/document/pepgrantvs.001.0011a

Benjamin, J. (1990). An outline of intersubjectivity: The development of recognition. *Psychoanalytic Psychology*, *7*, 3346.

Bering, J. (2013). *Perv: The sexual deviant in all of us.* Scientific American.

Bernard, P., Gervais, S., & Allen, J. (2012). Integrating sexual objectification with object versus person recognition: The sexualized body-inversion hypothesis. *Psychological Science*, *23*(5), 469–471. In Villarica, H. (2012). Study: The objectification of women is a real, measurable phenomenon. *The Atlantic*. May 24, 2012.

Bertrand, M., & Pan, J. (2013). The trouble with boys' social influences and the gender gap in disruptive behaviors. *American Economic Journal: Applied Economics*, pp. 32–64. In Schore, A. (2016). "All our sons: The developmental neurobiology and neuroendocrinology of boys at risk." *Infant Mental Health Journal*, 1–36.

Bion, W. (1961a). *Experiences in groups*. Tavistock.

Bion, W. (1961b). The psychoanalytic study of thinking. *International Journal of Psychoanalysis*, *43*, 306–310.

Bion, W. (1962). A theory of thinking. In E. Spillius (Ed.), *Melanie Klein today* (1988) (pp. 178–186). (vol. 1). Routledge.

Bion, W. (1967). Notes on memory and desire. *The Psychoanalytic Forum*, *2*, 272–273.

Bion, W. (1978). A Seminar in Paris. Held on July 10th. Transcribed by Francesca Bion.

Bion, W. R. (1959). Attacks on linking. *International Journal of Psychoanalysis*, *40*, 308–315.

Black, C. (2009). *Deceived*. Hazelden Publishing.

Blevins, J. W. (2016, November 12). How the concepts of "sex addiction" and "porn addiction" are failing our clients. *The Therapist*. California Association of Marriage & Family Therapists.

Bly, R. (1988). *A little book on the human shadow*. HarperOne.

Bly, R. (1990). *Iron John: A book about men*. Da Capo Press.

Bly, R. (1992). *What have I ever lost by dying?* HarperCollins.

Boszormenyi-Nagy, I. (1967). Relational modes and meaning. In G. H. Zuk & I. Boszormenyi-Nagy. *Family therapy and disturbed families*. Science and Behavior Books.

Boszormenyi-Nagy, I. (1972). Loyalty implications of the transference model in psychotherapy. *Archives of General Psychiatry*, *27*, 374–380.

Bowen, M. (1966). The use of family therapy in clinical practice. *Comprehensive Psychiatry*, 7, 345–374.

Bowlby, J. (1949). The study and reduction of group tension in the family. *Human Relations*, 2, 123–128.

Bowlby, J. (1960). Grief and mourning in infancy and early childhood. *The Psychoanalytic Study of the Child*, *15*, 9–53.

Braun-Harvey, D., & Vigorito, M. (2016). *Treating out of control sexual behavior: Rethinking sex addiction*. Springer.

Butler, M. (2010). Infidelity secrets in couple therapy: Therapists' views on the collision of competing ethics around relationship-relevant secrets. *Sexual Addiction & Compulsivity*, *17*, 82–105.

Carey, B. (2004, June 8). Pills or talk? If you're confused, no wonder. *New York Times*, https://www.nytimes.com/2004/06/08/health/pills-or-talk-if-you-re-confused-no-wonder.html

Carnes, P. (1989). *Contrary to love: Helping the sexual addict*. CompCare Publications.

Carnes, P. (1991). *Don't call it love*. Bantam Books.

Carnes, P. (2001). *Out of the shadows: Understanding sex addiction* (3rd ed.). Hazelden.

Carnes, S., Lee, M., & Rodriguez, A. D. (2012). *Facing heartbreak: Steps to recovery for partners of sex addicts*. Gentle Path Press.

Cermak, T. L. (1986). *Diagnosing and treating codependence*. Johnson Institute.

Coltart, N. (1987). Diagnosis and assessment for suitability for psycho-analytic psychotherapy. *British Journal of Psychotherapy*, *4*(2), 127–134.

Cooper, A., Delmonico, D., & Burg, R. (2000). Cybersex users, abusers, compulsives: New findings and implications. *Sexual Addiction & Compulsivity*, 7, 5–29.

Corey, G. (2008). *Theory and practice of group counseling* (7th ed.). Thomas Brooks/Cole.

Corley, D., Pollard, S., Hook, J., & Schneider, J. (2013). Impact of Disclosure of Relapse for Self-Identified Sex Addicts. *Sexual Addiction & Compulsivity*, *20*, 157–170.

Corley, M., & Schneider, J. (2002). Disclosing secrets: Guidelines for therapists working with sex addicts and co-addicts. *Sexual Addiction & Compulsivity*, *9*, 43–67. Brunner-Routledge.

Del Giudice, J., & Kutinsky, J. (2007). Applying motivational interviewing to the treatment of sexual compulsivity and addiction. *Sexual Addiction & Compulsivity*, *14*(4).

Diamond, M. J. (1997). The unbearable agony of being: Interpreting tormented states of mind in the psychoanalysis of sexually traumatized patients. *Bulletin of the Menninger Clinic*, *61*, 495–519.

Diamond, M. J. (2020). Treating the traumatized mind: Dissociation and psychoanalytic technique: the analyst's internal couple and maturing intimacy. *Psychoanalytic Quarterly*, *83*, 525–563.

Dickensen, J., Gleason, N., & Coleman, E. (2018). "Prevalence of distress associated with difficulty controlling sexual urges, feelings, and behaviors in the United States." *Journal of the American Medical Association*. November 9, 2018.

Dicks, H. V. (1967). *Marital Tensions*. Basic Books.

Dimberg, U., Thunberg, M., & Elmehed, K. (2000). Unconscious facial reactions to emotional facial expression. *Psychological Science*. Association for Psychological Science.

Director, L. (2002). The Value of Relational Psychoanalysis in the Treatment of Chronic Drug and Alcohol Use. *Psychoanalytic Dialogues*, *12*(4), 551–579.

Duncan, B. (2005). Treatment manuals do not improve outcomes. In J. C. Norcross. *Evidence-based practices in mental health: Debate and dialogue on the fundamental questions*. American Psychological Association Press.

Dworkin, R. (1991). "Liberty and Pornography." *New York Review of Books*, *XXXII*, 14.

Edmundson, M. (2007, September 9). Defender of the Faith? *New York Times Magazine*.

Eliot, L., Tan, A., Ma, W., Vira, A., & Marwha, D. (2015). The human hippocampus is not sexually dimorphic: Meta-analysis of structural MRI volumes. *Neuroimage*, *124*, 350–366.

Fairbairn, W. R. D. (1944). Endopsychic structure considered in terms of object relations. *International Journal of Psychoanalysis*, *25*, 70–92.

Farrell, W. (1999). *Women can't hear what men don't say*. Jeremy P. Tarcher/Penguin.

Ferenczi, S. (1930). The principle of relaxation and neocatharsis. *International Journal of Psychoanalysis*, *10*, 125–129.

Ferenczi, S. (1933). Confusion of tongues between adults and the child. In M. Balint (Ed.), C. Mosbacher (Trans.), *Final contributions to the problem and methods of psycho-analysis* (pp. 156–167). Karnac Books.

Ferguson, C. J., & Hartley, R. D. (2009). The pleasure is momentary . . . The expense damnable. *Aggression and Violent Behavior, 14*(5), 323–329.

Ferree, M. (Ed.). (2012). *Making advances: A comprehensive guide for treating female sex and love addicts*. Society for the Advancement of Sexual Health.

Fife, S. (2013). Facilitating forgiveness in the treatment of infidelity: An interpersonal model. *Journal of Family Therapy, 35*, 343–367.

Fincham, F. (2017). Infidelity in romantic relationships. *Current Opinion in Psychology, 13*, 70–74.

Fine, C. (2010). *Delusions of gender*. W. W. Norton.

Follette, V. M., Polusny, M. A., Bechtle, A. E., & Naugle, A. E. (1996). Cumulative trauma: The impact of child sexual abuse, adult sexual assault, and spouse abuse. *Journal of Traumatic Stress, 9*(1), 25–35.

Fonagy, P. (2008, March 1). A genuinely developmental theory of sexual enjoyment and its implications for psychoanalytic technique. *Journal of the American Psychoanalytic Association, 1*, 11–36.

Fonagy, P., & Target, M. (1996). Playing with reality: Theory of mind and the normal development of psychic reality. *International Journal of Psychoanalysis, 77*, 217–233.

Frazer, J. G. (1981). *The golden bough: The roots of religion and folklore*. Avenal Books. (Originally published in 1890)

Freud, S. (1894). The neuro-psychoses of defense. In *Standard Edition* (vol. 3) (pp. 45–61). Hogarth Press.

Freud, S. (1905). Three essays on the theory of sexuality. In *The standard edition of the complete works of Sigmund Freud*. (J. Strachey, Trans.) (vol. 16) (p. 80). In *Sexual Addiction & Compulsivity*. Hogarth Press.

Freud, S. (1909). Two case histories: Little Hans and the rat man. In *Standard Edition* (vol. 10). Hogarth Press.

Freud, S. (1911). Formulations on the two principles of mental functioning. In *Standard Edition* (vol. 12) (pp. 218–226). Hogarth Press.

Freud, S. (1912). The most prevalent form of degradation in erotic life. First published in *Jahrbuch* Bd. IV.

Freud, S. (1913). *Totem and taboo: Some points of agreement between the mental lives of savages and neurotics*. (J. Strachey, Ed. & Trans.). W. W. Norton.
Freud, S. (1914a). On narcissism: An introduction. In *Standard Edition* (vol. 14) (pp. 72–102). Hogarth Press.
Freud, S. (1914b). Remembering, repeating and working through. In *Standard Edition* (vol. 12) (pp. 145–156). Hogarth Press.
Freud, S. (1915). Repression. In *Standard Edition* (vol. 14) (pp. 141–158). Hogarth Press.
Freud, S. (1917). Mourning and melancholia. In *The standard edition of the complete psychological works of Sigmund Freud*. (J. Strachey, Trans.). Hogarth Press.
Freud, S. (1921). Group psychology and the analysis of the ego. In *The standard edition of the complete works of Sigmund Freud* (vol. 18). Hogarth Press.
Freud, S. (1923). The ego and the id. In *The standard edition of the complete psychological works of Sigmund Freud* (J. Strachey, Trans.). Hogarth Press.
Freud, S. (1924). The dissolution of the Oedipus complex. In *Standard Edition* (vol. 19) (pp. 173–179). Hogarth Press.
Freud, S. (1930). *Civilization and its discontents*. (J. Strachey, Ed. & Trans.). W. W. Norton.
Freud, S. (1933). *New introductory lectures on psychoanalysis*. W. W. Norton.
Freud, S. (2017). The psychopathology in everyday life. In A. A. Brill (Ed. & Trans.), *Collected Works of Sigmund Freud* (p. 1125). Delphi Classics. (Original work published 1901)
Freud, S., & Breuer, J. (1895). *Studies in hysteria, the standard edition of the complete psychological works of Sigmund Freud* (vol. 2). Hogarth Press and The Institute of Psychoanalysis.
Friedan, B. (1963). *The feminine mystique*. W. W. Norton.
Furman, E. (1992). On feeling and feeling felt. *Psychoanalytic Study of the Child*, *47*, 67–84.
Gao, S., Becker, B., & Kendrick, K. (2016, July 5). Oxytocin, the peptide that bonds the sexes also divides them. *Proceedings of the National Academy of Science USA*, *113* (27).
Garcia, F. D. (2016). A comprehensive review of psychotherapeutic treatment of sexual addiction. *Journal of Groups in Addiction & Recovery*, *11*(1), 59–71.
Gay, P. (1988). *Freud: A life for our time*. W. W. Norton.

Gilligan, C. (2010). Free association and the grand inquisitor: A drama in four acts. *Contemporary Psychoanalysis*, 6, 311–333.

Giugliano, J. (2006). Out of control sexual behavior: A qualitative investigation. *Sexual Addiction & Compulsivity*, *13*(4), 361–375.

Gladwell, M. (2008). *Outliers: The story of success*. Little, Brown, and Company.

Grubbs, J., Exline, J., Pargament, K., Hook, J. N., & Carlisle, R. (2014). Transgression as addiction: Religiosity and moral disapproval as predictors of perceived addiction to pornography. *Archives of Sexual Behavior*, *44*(1), 125–136.

Guntrip, H. (1969). *Schizoid phenomena: Object relations and the self*. International Universities Press.

Harlow, H. (1966). Effects of three months of total social deprivation on social adjustment and learning in the rhesus monkey. *Child Development*, *37*(3), 533–547.

Hentsch-Cowles, G., & Brock, L. J. (2013). A systemic review of the literature on the role of the partner of the sex addict, treatment models, and a call for research for systems theory model for treating the partner. *Sex Addiction & Compulsivity*, *20*(4), 323–335.

Holden, C. (2005). Sex and the suffering brain. *Science*, *308*, 1574–1577.

Holmes, G., Offen, L., & Waller, G. (1997). See no evil, hear no evil, speak no evil: Why do relatively few male victims of childhood sexual arousal receive help for abuse-related issues in adulthood? *Clinical Psychology Reviews*, *17*(1), 69–88.

Hook, J. N., Farrell, J. E., Davis, D. E., Van Tongeren, D. R., Griffin, B. J., Grubbs, J., & Bedics, J. D. (2015). Self-forgiveness and hypersexual behavior. *Sexual Addiction & Compulsivity*, *22*(1), 59–70.

Horney, K. (1924). On the genesis of the castration complex in women. *International Journal of Psychoanalysis*, *5*, 50–65.

Horney, K. (1926). The flight from womanhood: The masculinity complex in women, as viewed by men and by women. *International Journal of Psychoanalysis*, *7*, 324–339.

Hunt, S. A., & Kraus, S. W. (2009). Exploring the relationship between erotic disruption during the latency period and the use of sexually explicit material, online sexual behaviors, and sexual dysfunctions in young adulthood. *Sexual Addiction & Compulsivity*, *16*, 79–100.

Ikemata, S., & Panksepp, J. (1999). The role of nucleus accumbens dopamine in motivated behavior: A unifying interpretation with special reference to reward-seeking. *Brain Research and Brain Research Reviews*, *31*, 6–41.

Jacobs, T. (1986). On countertransference enactments. *Journal of the American Psychoanalytic Association*, *4*, 289–307.

Jagger, M., & Richards, K. (1969). You can't always get what you want. On *Let it bleed*. Olympic Studio.

Janet, P. (1889). *L'automatisme psychologique*. Felix Alcan.

Kalichman, S. C., & Rompa, D. (1995). Sexual sensation seeking and sexual compulsivity scales: Validity and predicting high-risk behavior. *Journal of Personality Assessment*, *65*(3), 586–601.

Kant, I. (2009). *An answer to the question: What is enlightenment?* Penguin Books. (Originally published in 1784)

Katehakis, A. (2009). Affective neuroscience and the treatment of sexual addiction. *Sexual Addiction & Compulsivity*, *16*, 1–31.

Katehakis, A. (2010). *Erotic Intelligence: Igniting hot, healthy sex while in recovery from sex addiction*. Health Communications, Inc.

Katehakis, A. (2016). From victimhood to victorhood: Treating partners of sex addicts. *The Therapist*, *27*(3): 6–9.

Kelly, R. J., Wood, J. J., Gonzalez, L., MacDonald, V., & Waterman, J. (2002). Effects of mother-son incest and positive perceptions of sexual abuse experiences on the psychosocial adjustment of clinic-referred men. *Child Abuse & Neglect*, *26*(4), 425–441.

Khantzian, E. J. (1981). Some treatment implications of the ego and self disturbances in alcoholism. In M. H. Bean & N. E. Zinberg (Eds.), *Dynamic approaches to the understanding and treatment of alcoholism* (pp. 163–188). Free Press.

Klaassen, M., & Peter, J. (2015). Gender inequality in internet pornography: A content analysis of popular pornographic internet videos. *Journal of Sex Research*, *52*(7), 721–735.

Klein, M. (1928). Early stages of Oedipal complex. *International Journal of Psychoanalysis*, *9*, 167–180.

Klein, M. (1935). A contribution to the psychogenesis of manic-depressive states. In *Contributions to psychoanalysis, 1921–1945*. McGraw-Hill.

Klein, M. (1940). Mourning and its relation to manic-depressive states. In *Contributions to psychoanalysis, 1921–1945*. McGraw-Hill.

Klein, M. (1946). Notes of some schizoid mechanisms. *International Journal of Psychoanalysis*, *27*, 99–110.

Klein, M. (2012, July/August). You're addicted to what? Challenging the myth of sex addiction. *Humanist*. http://thehumanist.com/july-august-2012/you're-addicted-to-what/

Kohut, H. (1971). *The analysis of the self: A systematic approach to the psychoanalytic treatment of narcissistic personality disorders*. International Universities Press.

Kohut, H. (1977). Preface to *Psychodynamics of drug dependence*. National Institute on Drug Abuse Research Monograph #12.

Kort, J. (2015). Why I am no longer a sex addiction therapist. *The Good Man Project*. http://goodmanproject.com/featured-content/why-I-am-no-longer-a-sex-addiction-therapist/

Kristeva, J. (1974). *Revolution in poetic language* (M. Waller, Trans.). Colombia University Press.

Lacan, J. (1938). Family complexes in the formation of the individual. *La Famille, Encyclopedie Francaise*.

Lacan, J. (1953). The neurotic's individual myth. *Psychoanalytic Quarterly*, *48*, 405–421.

Langton, R. (1993). Beyond a pragmatic critique of reason. *Australasian Journal of Philosophy*, *71*(4), 364–384.

Lazarus, A. (1994). A proposal for psychiatric collaboration in managed care. *American Journal of Psychotherapy*, *48*(4), 600–609.

Levy, A. (2005). *Female chauvinist pigs: Women and the rise of raunch culture*. Free Press.

Ley, D. (2012). *The myth of sex addiction*. Rowman & Littlefield.

Linden, D. J. (2011). *The compass of pleasure*. Viking.

Linehan, M., Chen, E., Brown, M., & Lo, T. (2007). Sexually transmitted disease rates and high risk sexual behaviors in borderline personality disorder versus borderline personality disorder with substance use disorder. *Journal of Nervous and Mental Disease*, *195*, 125–129.

Loewald, H. W. (1979). The waning of the Oedipus complex. *Journal of the American Psychoanalytic Association*, *27*, 751–775.

Lyons-Ruth, K. (2005). The two-person unconscious: Intersubjective dialogue, enactive relational representation, and the emergence of new forms of relational organization. In L. Aron & A. Harris (Eds.), *Relational Psychoanalysis* (vol. 2) (pp. 311–353). Analytic Press.

MacKinnon, C. (1987). *Feminism unmodified.* Cambridge University Press.

Madigan, S. (2018). Prevalence of multiple forms of sexting behavior among youth: A systematic review and meta-analysis. *JAMA Pediatrics, 172*(4), 327–335.

Mahler, M. (1975). *The psychological birth of the human infant.* Basic Books.

Main, M. (2000). The organized categories of infant, child, and adult attachment flexible vs. inflexible attention under attachment-related stress. *Journal of the American Psychoanalytic Association, 48*, 1055–1095.

Main, M., & Solomon, J. (1986). Discovery of an insecure-disorganized/disoriented attachment patter, pp. 95–124. In T. B. Brazelton & M. W. Yogman (Eds.), *Affective development in infancy*. Ablex Publishing.

Markale, J. (1972). *Women of the Celts.* Inner Traditions International, Ltd.

Marks-Tarlow, T. (2012). *The interpersonal neurobiology of clinical intuition in psychotherapy*. W. W. Norton.

Masterson, J. (1976). *Psychotherapy of the borderline adult: A developmental approach*. Brunner/Mazel.

Masterson, J. (1981). *The narcissistic and borderline disorders: An integrated developmental approach*. Brunner/Mazel.

Masterson, J. (1985). *The real self: A developmental, self, and object relations approach*. Brunner/Mazel.

Masterson, J. (1988). *The search for the real self: Unmasking the personality disorders of our age.* Free Press.

Masterson, J. (2000). *The personality disorders: A New look at the developmental self and object relations approach*. Zeig, Tucker & Co.

Masterson, J. F., & Klein, R. (1995). *Disorder of the self: New therapeutic horizons, the Masterson approach*. Brunner/Mazel.

Mathews, D. (2019). Personal communication.

Mayer, E. L. (1985). "Everybody must be just like me": Observations on female castration anxiety. *International Journal of Psychoanalysis*, 66, 331–347.

Meares, R. (2012). *A dissociation model of borderline personality disorder*. W. W. Norton.

Melody, P. (1989). *Facing codependence: What it is, where it comes from, how it sabotages our lives*. HarperSanFrancisco.

Miller, W. R., & Rollnick, S. (2002). *Motivational interviewing: Preparing people for change*. Guilford Press.

Minuchin, S. (1974). *Families and family therapy*. Harvard University Press.

Minwalla, O. (2012, July 23). Partners of sex addicts need treatment for trauma. *The National Psychologist*.

Minwalla, O. (2017). Sex addiction induced trauma and its 13 dimensions. https://togetherwecanheal.com/sex-addiction-induced-trauma-how-sex-addiction-impacts-the-partners/#top

Mitrani, J. L. (2001). Taking the transference: Some technical implications in three papers by Bion. *International Journal of Psychoanalysis*, *82*, 1085.

Moore, T. (2009). *Care of the soul: Guide for cultivating depth and sacredness in everyday life*. HarperCollins.

Moss, D. (2019). Free speech, love speech, hate speech, and neutrality: In and out of the consulting room. *Journal of the American Psychoanalytic Association*, *67*, 2.

Myers, W. A. (1995). Addictive sexual behavior. *American Journal of Psychotherapy*, *49*, 473–483.

Nayoung, L. (2010, June). Individual and work-related factors influencing burnout of mental health professionals: A meta-analysis. *Journal of Employment Counseling*, 92–93.

Nowak, C. (2019). *11 monogamous animals that stay together all of their lives*. Readers Digest.

Nowell, E. (1960). *Thomas Wolfe: A biography*. Doubleday.

Nussbaum, M. (1995). Objectification. *Philosophy and Public Affairs*, *24*(4), 249–291.

Ogden, T. (2005). *This art of psychoanalysis: Dreaming undreamt dreams and interrupted cries*. Routledge.

Ogden, T. H. (1989). *The primitive edge of experience*. Jason Aronson.

Opitz, D. M., Tsytsarev, S. V., & Froh, J. (2009). Women's sexual addiction and family dynamics, depression and substance abuse. *Sexual Addiction & Compulsivity*, *16*, 324–340.

Osborne, T. (2015, August 7). New research sheds light on sex abuse committed by mothers against their sons. ABC News. https://

www.abc.net.au/news/2015-08-08/new-research-mothers-who-sexually-abuse-their-sons/6679102
Perel, E (2006). *Mating in captivity: Unlocking erotic intelligence.* HarperCollins.
Perel, E. (2017). *State of affairs: Rethinking infidelity.* Harper.
Pinker, S. (2012). *The better angels of our nature: Why violence has declined.* Penguin.
Potenza, M. N. (2006). Should addictive disorders include non-substance-related conditions? *Addiction, 101*(Suppl. 1), 142–151.
Real, T. (1998). *I don't want to talk about it.* Scribner.
Real, T. (2003). *How can I get through to you.* Fireside.
Redford, R. (Director). (1998). *The horse whisperer [Film].* Touchstone Pictures.
Reid, R., Carpenter, B., Garos, S., & Najavits, L. (2013). Personality disorder comorbidity in treatment-seeking men with hypersexual disorder. *Sexual Addiction & Compulsivity, 20*, 79–90.
Reid, R., Kor, A., Fogel, Y., & Potenza, M. (2013). Should hypersexual disorder be classified as an addiction? *Sexual Addiction & Compulsivity, 20*, 27–47.
Riviere, J. (1936). A contribution to the analysis of the negative therapeutic reaction. *International Journal of Psycho-Analysis, 17*, 304–320.
Roberts, D. (2007). *Another chance to be real: Attachment and object relations treatment of borderline personality disorder.* Jason Aronson.
Rosenberg, T. (2006, January). Burnout among mental health professionals: Special considerations for the marriage and family therapist. *Journal of Marital and Family Therapy, 32*(1), 87–99.
Ryan, C., & Jetha, C. (2010). *Sex at dawn: The prehistoric origins of modern sexuality.* Harper Perennial.
Sansone, R., Chu, J., & Wiederman, M. W. (2011). Sexual behavior and borderline personality disorder among female psychiatric inpatients. *International Journal of Psychiatry in Clinical Practice, 15*, 69–73.
Santorelli, S. (1999). *Heal thy self: Lessons on mindfulness in medicine.* Harmony.
Schore, A. (2010). Attachment trauma and the developing right brain: Origins of pathological dissociation. In P. Dell (Ed.), *Dissociation and the dissociative disorders: DSM-V and beyond* (pp. 107–129). Routledge.

Schore, A. N. (1994). *Affect regulation and the origin of the self: The neurobiology of emotional development*. Erlbaum.
Schore, A. N. (2000, January). Clinical implications of a psychoneurobiological model of projective identification. *Infant Observation, 3*(3), 91–93.
Schore, A. N. (2016). All our sons: The developmental neurobiology and neuroendocrinology of boys at risk. *Infant Mental Health Journal, 38*(1), 1–36.
Seligman, L., & Hardenburg, S. A. (2000). Assessment and treatment of paraphilias. *Journal of Counseling & Development, 78*(1), 107–114.
Seto, M., Hanson, R., & Babchishin, K. (2011). Contact sexual offending by men with online sexual offenses. *Sexual Abuse: A Journal of Research & Treatment, 23*(1), 124–145.
Shafron-Perez, S. (2009). Average teenager or sex offender? Solutions to the legal dilemma caused by sexting. *The John Marshall Journal of Computer & Information Law*, 26.
Shedler, J. (2010). The efficacy of psychodynamic psychotherapy. *American Psychologist, 65*(2), 98–109.
Siegel, D. (1999). *The developing mind*. Guildford Press.
Siegel, D. (2012). *The developing mind: How relationships and the brain interact to shape who we are* (2nd ed.). Guilford Press.
Silverstein, J. (1998). Countertransference in marital therapy for infidelity. *Journal of Sex and Marital Therapy, 24*, 293–301.
Skinner, K. B. (2015, August). The lasting effects of sexual betrayal. *Psychology Today*. https://www.psychologytoday.com/us/blog/inside-porn-addiction/201508/the-powerful-and-lasting-effects-sexual-betrayal
Solnit, R. (2020). *Recollections of my nonexistence*. Viking.
Sontag, S. (1973). *On photography*. Picador.
Stafford, W. (1998). *The way it is: New and selected poems*. Graywolf Press.
Steffens, B., & Means, M. (2009). *Your sexually addicted spouse*. New Horizons Press.
Steffens, B., & Rennie, R. (2006). The traumatic nature of disclosure for the wives of sexual addicts. *Sexual Addiction & Compulsivity, 13*, 247–267.
Stemple, L., & Meyer, I. (2017, December). Sexual victimization by women is more common than previously known. *Scientific American Mind, 29*(1): 54–57.

Stokes, S., Moulton, S., Sudweeks, R. R., & Fischer, L. (2020). An item analysis of the trauma inventory for partners of sex addicts. *Sexual Addiction & Compulsivity*, *27*(1–2).

Stoller, R. J. (1968). *Sex and gender* (vol. 1). Science House.

Stone, M. (2006). The analyst's body as tuning fork: Embodied resonance in countertransference. *Journal of Analytical Psychology*, *51*(1), 109–124.

Sussman, S. (2010). Love addiction: Definition, etiology, treatment. *Sexual Addiction & Compulsivity*, *17*(1), 31–45.

Terkel, S. (1974). *Working: People talk about what they do all day and how they feel about what they do*. Pantheon/Random House.

Tripodi, C. (2006). Long-term treatment of partners of sex addicts: A multi-phase approach. *Sexual Addiction & Compulsivity*, *13*(2–3), 269–288.

Van der Kolk, B., McFarlane, A., & Weisath, I. (Eds.). (1996). *Traumatic stress: The effects of overwhelming experience on mind, body, and society*. Guilford Press.

Voon, V., Mole, T., Banca, P., Porter, L., Morris, L., Mitchell, S., Lapa, T., Karr, J., Harrison, N., Potenza, M, & Irvine, M. (2014). Neural correlates of sexual cue reactivity in individuals with or without sexual compulsive behaviors. *PloS ONE*, *9* (7): e102419. https://doi.org/10.1371/journal.pone.0102419

Waska, R. (2006). Addictions and the quest for control of the object. *American Journal of Psychoanalysis*, *66*, 43.

Weiss, R. (2013). *Sex addiction 101: A basic guide to healing from sex, porn, and love addiction*. Telemachus Press.

Winnicott, D. W. (1952). Anxiety associated with insecurity. In D. W. Winnicott (Ed.), *Collected papers: Through paediatrics to psychoanalysis*, pp. 97–101. Routledge.

Winnicott, D. W. (1960). Ego distortion in terms of true and false self. In D. W. Winnicott (Ed.), *The maturational processes and the facilitating environment: Studies in the theory of emotional development* (pp. 140–152). Karnac Books

Winnicott, D. W. (Ed.) (1965). *The maturational processes and the facilitating environment: Studies in the theory of emotional development*. International Universities Press.

Winnicott, D. W. (1971). *Playing and reality*. Routledge.

Woehler, E., Giordano, A., & Hagedorn, B. (2018). Moments of relational depth in sex addiction treatment. *Sexual Addiction & Compulsivity*, *25*(2–3), 153–169.

Wolf, J. L. (2000). Assessment and treatment of compulsive sex/love behavior. *Journal of Rational-Emotive & Cognitive-Behavior Therapy*, *18*(4), 235–246.

World Health Organization. (2019). *International classification of diseases* (11th ed.). (ICD-11). WHO.

Yalom, I. (1995). *The theory and practice of group psychotherapy* (4th ed.). Basic Books.

Yeomans, F., Hull, J. W., & Clarkin, J. F. (1993). Borderline personality disorder and impulsive sexual behavior. *Hospital & Community Psychiatry*, *44*, 1000–1002.

Zanarini, M. C., Williams, A. A., & Lewis, R. E. (1997). Reported pathological childhood experiences associated with the development of borderline personality disorder. *American Journal of Psychiatry*, *154*, 1101–1106.

Zhou, Y. (2017, November 4). Goodreads data show that women reading self-help books are getting advice from men. https://qz.com/1106341/most-women-reading-self-help-books-are-getting-advice-from-men/

Zitzman, S. T., & Butler, M. H. (2009). Wives' experience of husbands' pornography use and concomitant deception as an attachment threat in the adult pair-bond relationship. *Sexual Addiction & Compulsivity*, *16*, 210–240.

Index

About the Authors

Graeme Daniels, MFT, has been a practicing psychotherapist since 1996, working with individuals, couples, and groups, and treating a variety of mental health conditions, in hospital and private practice settings. Since 2011, he has been a prolific author, writing and self-publishing several novels, and writing articles for online resources like PsycheCentral.com, as well as his own blog at www.selfinaddiction.com. In 2016, he wrote an 8,000-word academic article about OR theory and the rock opera *Tommy*, which was published within the *Journal of Culture and Psychology*, a Sage publication. His subsequent nonfiction book, *The Psychology of Tommy*, made the Kirkus Reviews Indie book of the month list in 2019. He has made professional presentations at the 2015 SASH conference in San Diego and at the 2017 and 2021 "Creativity and Madness" conferences in Santa Fe, New Mexico. Concurrently, he provides trainings at San Francisco Bay Area mental health agencies on the Disorder of Self model of Dr. James Masterson and is a current faculty member within the Masterson Institute, as well as an analytic training candidate within the San Francisco Center for Psychoanalysis.

Joseph P. Farley, MFT, is a marriage and family therapist in private practice in Walnut Creek, California. He was appointed to the faculty of the Masterson Institute for Psychoanalytic Psychotherapy in 2002 and as the Clinical Director in 2007. James Masterson chose him as one of two heirs to run his institute after his death. Farley has over 35 years of clinical experience in working with adolescents, couples, and individual adults. He has also taught at the graduate psychology department at John F. Kennedy University and lectured at The Wright Institute, Alliant University, University of California, Berkeley, and Vancouver Island University. His chapter, "Nice Guys Finish Last," was included in Dr. Masterson's final publication as editor, *The Personality Disorders Through the Lens of Attachment Theory and the Neurobiologic Development of the Self* in 2005.

www.ingramcontent.com/pod-product-compliance
Ingram Content Group UK Ltd.
Pitfield, Milton Keynes, MK11 3LW, UK
UKHW021904150926
475560UK00004B/336

9 781538 158043